Panda's

Practical
Prescriber

with Differential Diagnosis

Panda's Practical Prescriber

with Differential Diagnosis

U.N. PANDA MD

Senior Consultant (Medicine)
New Delhi

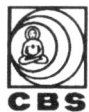

CBS

CBS Publishers & Distributors Pvt. Ltd.

New Delhi • Bengaluru • Chennai • Kochi • Kolkata • Mumbai
Hyderabad • Uttarakhand • Nagpur • Patna • Pune • Jharkhand

Practical Prescriber
with Differential Diagnosis

ISBN: 81-239-1204-8

First Edition: 2005
Reprint: 2006, 2016, 2018

Copyright © 2005, Author & Publisher

All rights reserved. No part of this book may be reproduced or transmitted in any form or by any means, electronic or mechanical, including photocopying, recording, or any information storage and retrieval system without permission, in writing, from the publisher.

Published by **Satish Kumar Jain** and produced by **Varun Jain** for
CBS Publishers & Distributors Pvt. Ltd.,
4819/XI Prahlad Street, 24 Ansari Road, Daryaganj, New Delhi - 110002
delhi@cbspd.com, cbspubs@airtelmail.in • www.cbspd.com
Ph.: 23289259, 23266861, 23266867 • Fax: 011-23243014

Corporate Office: 204 FIE, Industrial Area, Patparganj, Delhi - 110 092
Ph: 49344934 • Fax: 011-49344935
E-mail: publishing@cbspd.com • publicity@cbspd.com

Branches:
• *Bengaluru:* 2975, 17th Cross, K.R. Road, Bansankari 2nd Stage, Bengaluru - 70 • Ph: +91-80-26771678/79 • Fax: +91-80-26771680
E-mail: cbsbng@gmail.com, bangalore@cbspd.com
• *Chennai:* No. 7, Subbaraya Street, Shenoy Nagar, Chennai - 600030
Ph: +91-44-26681266, 26680620 • Fax: +91-44-42032115
E-mail: chennai@cbspd.com
• *Kochi:* Ashana House, 39/1904, A.M. Thomas Road, Valanjambalam, Ernakulum, Kochi • Ph: +91-484-4059061-65
Fax: +91-484-4059065 • E-mail: cochin@cbspd.com
• *Kolkata:* 6-B, Ground Floor, Rameshwar Shaw Road, Kolkata - 700014
Ph: +91-33-22891126/7/8 • E-mail: kolkata@cbspd.com
• *Mumbai:* 83-C, Dr. E. Moses Road, Worli, Mumbai - 400018
Ph: +91-9833017933, 022-24902340/41 • E-mail: mumbai@cbspd.com

Representatives:

• Hyderabad: 0-9885175004	• Nagpur: 0-9021734563
• Patna: 0-9334159340	• Pune: 0-9623451994
• Jharkhand: 0-9811541605	• Uttarakhand: 0-9716462459

Printed at:
India Binding House, Noida, UP (India)

dedicated

to

my wife
Chinmoyee

and

my sons
Santosh and
Shashwat

Preface

In today's busy medical practice the doctor has hardly enough time to consult or confer. He has to task his memory for diagnosis, investigation and treatment. A fatigued memory often does not oblige easily. To overcome this a handbook providing easy access to diagnosis, investigation and treatment is very helpful.

Practical Prescriber with Differential Diagnosis is a humble work in this direction depicting the salient features of common diseases encountered in day-to-day practice. The book only provides direction but not minute details. The tables help to identify one disease that closely mimics another. The *Prescriber* is expected to be of immense help to busy practitioners as well as interns and residents who can use it for quick reference.

All suggestions for improvement are welcome.

Dr. U.N. PANDA
Senior Consultant (Medicine)
New Delhi

Contents

2 Renal Diseases 45

3 Endocrine Disorders 59

4 Diseases of Lungs and Respiration 79

5 Cardiovascular Diseases 103

6 Nervous System 121

7 Diseases of Alimentary Tract 149

8 Hepatobiliary Diseases 171

9 Diseases of Blood 185

10 Rheumatic Disorders 199

11 Electrolyte Disorders 207

12 Skin Diseases 213

13 Poisoning 223

14 Psychiatric Disorders 229

Appendices 239

Index 259

Panda's
Practical
Prescriber
with Differential Diagnosis

1

INFECTIOUS DISEASES

HERPES SIMPLEX

Essentials of diagnosis

- Herpes simplex viruses cause primary disease as well as reactivation.
- HSV I causes herpes labial is involving lips and oral cavity, whitlows, keratoconjunctivitis, dendritic corneal ulcer, Bell's palsy, meningoencephalitis, esophagitis, erythema-multiforme.
- HSV II causes infection of genital tract with multiple painful, small, grouped vesicles.
- Direct fluorescent antibody staining of scrapping from lesion/PCR are diagnostic.

Treatment

- Trifluridine 1% drops every 2 hours for HSV keratitis.
- Topical 5% acyclovir ointment for mucocutaneous disease.
- Oral acyclovir 200 mg 5 times daily for genital infection.
- Acyclovir 5–10 mg/kg IV every 8 hours for esophagitis, encephalitis and disseminated neonatal disease.
- In immunocompromised foscarnet 20 mg/kg IV twice daily with gradual reduction.
- AIDS patients with history of mucocutaneous disease should receive life-long acyclovir suppression.
- Patients of recurrent genital herpes/mucocutaneous disease should receive acyclovir 400 mg bid/famciclovir 250 mg bid or valacyclovir 500 mg bid as prophylaxis.

CHICKENPOX AND HERPES ZOSTER

Essentials of diagnosis

- Fever, malaise (more so in adults).
- Vesicular eruptions (may appear first in oropharynx), prominent on face and trunk, sparse on limbs.
- Rapid conversion of pruritic rash to vesicles, pustules and crusting stage.
- New eruptions occur every 1–5 days; hence all stages of eruption are present simultaneously.
- Pain precedes appearance of rash in HZ and follows nerve root distribution. When lesions occur on the tip of nose, corneal involvement is likely.
- Geniculate ganglion involvement (Ramsay-Hunt syndrome) causes facial palsy, lesions in external ear, vertigo, tinnitus and deafness.
- Varicella may be complicated by interstitial pneumonia, pulmonary calcification, ARDs, hepatitis, Reye's syndrome (hepatitis with encephalopathy), Bell's palsy.
- Postherpetic neuralgia occurs in 50% cases if over 60 years.

Treatment

- Isolation till crusts fall off.
- Topical calamine lotion, antihistaminics to relieve pruritus.
- Antiviral therapy (acyclovir, valacyclovir, famciclovir) if immunocompromised or to shorten duration and severity of attack, both chickenpox and zoster (acyclovir 800 mg 5 times daily).
- Short course of steroid treatment may prevent postherpetic neuralgia but is not routinely indicated.
- Prevention is by live attenuated varicella vaccine to those above 12 months of age without having suffered from chickenpox. A second dose after 1–2 months of first dose is recommended for adults.
- Exposed susceptibles be given VZIG 12.5 units/kg.

INFECTIOUS MONONUCLEOSIS

Essentials of diagnosis

- Malaise, fever, sore throat, cervical lymphadenopathy (posterior chain).
- Maculopapular rash (occasional), splenomegaly (in 50%), petechiae on soft palate.
- Occasionally hepatitis, mononeuropathy, meningo-encephalitis, pneumonitis, myocarditis, interstitial nephritis, etc.
- Atypical lymphocytosis positive (darkly staining, large, foamy).
- Positive neutrophil antibody or monospot test (within 4 weeks of illness).

Treatment

- Symptomatic relief with NSAIDs.
- Penciclovir (prodrug of famciclovir) may be effective.
- Death can occur due to splenic rupture or hypersplenism (severe haemolytic anaemia, thrombocytopenia) or encephalitis but are very rare.

CMV INFECTION

Essentials of diagnosis

- Perinatal disease, acquired in utero; is characterised by hepatosplenomegaly, jaundice, CNS calcification, motor disability and purpura.
- Acute acquired CMV resembles infectious mononucleosis but with leukopenia and negative monospot test.
- Disease in immunocompromised causes CMV retinitis, (pizza – pie retinopathy), colitis, pulmonary disease, transverse myelitis – encephalitis.
- PCR and viral culture are diagnostic.

Treatment

- Ganciclovir 5 mg/kg IV twice daily for 14–21 days or cidofovir 5 mg/kg IV every week for 2 weeks or foscarnet IV followed by maintenance with daily ganciclovir once IV or cidofovir every 2 weeks.
- Resistant strains need fomivirsen, an anti HIV agent.

MEASLES

Essentials of diagnosis

- Prodrome of fever, cough, coryza, conjunctivitis, Koplik's spots.
- Brick red irregular maculopapular rash, beginning in face and affecting soles and palms last, appear 3–4 days after the prodrome.
- Leucopenia
- Atypical measles in adults causes high fever, papular-haemorrhagic rash without Koplik's spots, hepatitis, interstitial pneumonitis.
- Complications include encephalitis (acute/subacute), bronchopneumonia, protein loosing enteropathy (often preceded by rectal Koplik's spots).

Treatment

- Symptomatic with isolation and bed rest.
- Vitamin A, 4 lac units daily orally to enhance mucosal immunity and integrity.
- Prevention is by live attenuated measles vaccine, one dose at 9–12 months and second at 4–5 years.

MUMPS

Essentials of diagnosis

- Painful swollen salivary glands, usually the parotids.

- Often there is orchitis, oophoritis, pancreatitis and meningitis.
- Relative lymphocytosis.
- Rare complications are encephalitis, nephritis, myocarditis, hepatitis.

Treatment

- Purely symptomatic with NSAID.
- Suspensory bandage, ice bags, painkillers or even procaine injection to spermatic cord for orchitis; hydrocortisone 100 mg IV followed by 20 mg orally every 6 hours for 2 days.
- Prevention is by vaccination (MMR vaccine).

POLIOMYELITIS

Essentials of diagnosis

- *Abortive Polio* – fever, diarrhea, sore throat.
- *Non Paralytic Polio* – above symptoms plus aseptic meningitis often with muscle spasm.
- *Paralytic Poliomyelitis* – (a) spinal form – paralysis of muscles innervated by spinal nerves (b) bulbar polio – paralysis of cranial nerves particularly 9 and 10, vasomotor and respiratory centres.
- Atelectasis, pneumonia, myocarditis; respiratory muscle palsy may complicate.
- Post poliomyelitis syndrome – new muscle weakness after years of recovery from paralytic polio.

Treatment

- Complete bed rest.
- Polio bed (firm mattress, foot board, sand bags, light splints).
- Management of complication like respiratory palsy.
- Prevention by OPV 2 doses 4–6 weeks apart.

RUBELLA

Essentials of diagnosis

- Posterior cervical and post auricular lymphadenopathy.
- Fine maculopapular rash of 3 days duration from face to trunk to extremity.
- Arthralgia particularly in young women.
- Mild fever, coryza coinciding with eruption.
- Congenital rubella — psyohomotor retardation, congenital heart disease, microphthalmia.
- Post infectious encephalopathy (20% fatality) rarely.

Treatment

- Symptomatic
- Energetic treatment of encephalitis and thrombocytopenia.
- Prevention is by line attenuated vaccine (MMR) to children and susceptible girls before menarche.

RABIES

Essentials of diagnosis

- History of animal bite.
- Paresthesia, hydrophobia, rage alternating with calm.
- Convulsions, thick tenacious saliva.
- Fluorescent antibody staining of corneal impression.

Treatment

- Isolation and barrier nursing.
- Control of convulsion, maintenance of airway, and oxygenation.
- Prevention is by (a) preexposure prophylaxis with 3 doses of ARV at days A 0,7,21 (b) post-

exposure prophylaxis with 5 doses of ARV at days 0, 3, 7, 14, 28.

DENGUE

Essentials of diagnosis

• Sudden onset of high fever, chill, body pain, headache and sore throat.
• Biphasic rash — first evanescent followed by maculopapular, scarlantiniform, morbiliform or petechial.
• Biphasic fever curve — initial phase of 3–4 days; then remission for up to 2 days, then second phase of 1–2 days.
• Leukopenia and thrombocytopenia in the haemorrhagic forms (*Dengue Haemorrhagic Fever*).
• Sudden fatal shock (dengue shock syndrome), particularly in children.
• Expression of CD 69 on lymphocytes correlates with development of dengue haemorrhagic fever.
• Complications include pneumonia, bone marrow failure, orchitis-oophoritis.

Treatment

• Symptomatic treatment with NSAIDs.
• Fluid management and vasopressors for dengue shock syndrome.
• Platelet infusion for dengue haemorrhagic fever.

HANTAVIRUS SYNDROME

• Non-specific febrile illness progressing rapidly to shock, thrombocytopenia, increased pulmonary vascular permeability and ARDS (Hantavirus pulmonary syndrome).

- *Treatment* is symptomatic; ribavirin IV is helpful. 33 mg/kg loading then 16 mg/kg 4 times daily for 4 days and 8 mg/kg IV for next 3 days.

SEVERE ACUTE RESPIRATORY SYNDROME (SARS)

- Non specific febrile illness progressing rapidly to dyspnoea and hypoxemia with pulmonary interstitial infiltrates; mortality 4–10%.
- *Treatment* is symptomatic and that of respiratory failure.

YELLOW FEVER

- Sudden severe headache, bodyache and tachycardia.
- After a day of remission there is bradycardia, jaundice, proteinuria, hypotension, haemorrhagic tendency.
- History of exposure in endemic areas (Not in Asia).
- *Treatment* is symptomatic.

EBOLA-MARBURG DISEASE

- Fever with haemorrhage and rash due to thrombocytopenia.
- Rapid progression and early high fatality.
- *Treatment* is symptomatic with blood transfusion and control of shock and renal failure.
- Ribavirin as for Hantavirus may be worth trying.

RESPIRATORY SYNCYTIAL VIRUS

- Features of bronchiolitis, tracheobronchitis and pneumonia in very young. Proliferation and necrosis of bronchial epithelium causes obstruction, hyperinflation of lungs.
- *Treatment* is hydration, humidification of inspired air, antibiotic prophylaxis for secondary lung infection.

- Hyperimmune RSV IG 750 mg/kg every month to those with frequent attacks.
- Aerosolized ribavirin 1.1 g/d, diluted to 20 mg/ml delivered with oxygen over 12 hours daily for 3–7 days to those with underlying cardiopulmonary disease.
- Monoclonal antibody against RSV (palivizumab) is also available.

INFLUENZA

Essentials of diagnosis

- Abrupt onset of fever, chill, coryza and muscle ache; but fever and prostration are out of proportion to catarrhal symptoms.
- Leucopenia, flushed face, conjunctival congestion and pharyngeal injection.
- Secondary bacterial infection of respiratory tract is common leading to pneumonia, purulent bronchitis, sinusitis, otitis media, etc.
- *Reye's Syndrome* (fatty liver with encephalopathy) is a rare but fatal complication.

Treatment

- Bed rest, analgesics, cough suppressants.
- Amantadine or rimantadine 100 mg twice daily decrease the duration of disease. Alternatively zanamivir 5 mg inhalation twice daily or oseltamivir 75 mg PO twice daily.
- Chemoprophylaxis is also with above drugs in similar doses.

TYPHUS FEVERS

- High pronged fever, severe headache, chills, often leading to stupor.

- Macular rash appears on 4th to 7th day but spares face, palms and soles.
- Proteinuria and haematuria are common; hearing loss may occur, splenomegaly is not unusual so also patchy pneumonitis.
- In scrub typhus black eschar at site of mite bite, regional and generalised lymphadenopathy often complicated with encephalitis, pneumonitis, hepatitis, renal and cardiac failure.
- Brill's disease (recrudescent epidemic typhus) has more gradual course, fever and rash of shorter duration.
- Weil-Felix reaction is positive.
- All rickettsiae respond to doxycycline, tetracycline, chloramphenicol for 7 days; resistant cases, children and pregnant ladies be given azithromycin 250 mg bid for 7 days.

Q FEVER

- An acute or chronic febrile illness with severe headache, prostration, dry cough and abdominal pain.
- Extensive pneumonitis, granulomatous hepatitis, and rarely myocarditis, haemolytic anaemia, encephalo-pathy, mediastinal lymphadenopathy, orchitis, acute renal failure.
- Diagnosis is by rising complement fixing antibodies.
- *Treatment* is with doxycycline or tetracycline for 7 days. But in endocarditis treatment is with doxycycline or rifampicin (900 mg/d), fluoroquinolones and hydroxy-chloroquine, continued often for years.

KAWASAKI SYNDROME

- Otherwise known as mucocutaneous lymphnode syndrome with high vulnerability for Asian children.
- Characterised by fever, and four of the following for at least 5 days — bilateral nonexudative conjunctivitis,

injected pharynx/strawberry tongue, a polymorphous rash, cervical lymphadenopathy and extremity changes (edema, erythema, desquamation).
- Can be complicated by coronary arteritis myocardial infarction.
- Treatment is with aspirin 80–100 mg/kg/day.
- IVIG, plasmapheresis and corticosteroid can be beneficial.

STREPTOCOCCAL INFECTION

- Can cause pharyngitis, skin infections, arthritis, scarlet fever, pneumonia and empyema, endocarditis, necrotizing fascitis and toxic shock syndrome. Gram positive cocci are seen in smear.
- In pharyngitis there is fever, throat pain and headache; throat is red and edematous with tender cervical nodes; can be complicated by sinusitis, mastoiditis, rheumatic fever, glomerulonephritis. Treatment is with benzathine penicillin 1.2 MU IM single dose or azithromycin 500 mg daily for 3 days.
- Skin infections include impetigo (vesicopustular lesion with thick amber coloured crust) and erysipelas (spreading painful cellulitis). If patient is toxic treatment is with nafcillin 1.5 gm IV 6 hrly or vancomycin 1 gm IV bid, else amoxycillin 500 mg tid or cephalexin 500 mg qid for 5–7 days are sufficient.
- In septic arthritis Penicillin G, 2 MU every 4 hours with frequent percutaneous needle aspiration be done.
- IV penicillin with drainage be done in empyema.
- Group A streptococcal endocarditis involves tricuspid valve and be treated by penicillin G, 4 MU, 4 hourly for 4 weeks.
- In necrotising fascitis severe pain, systemic toxicity, compression of nerve and vessels are characteristic demanding surgical exploration and heavy doses of penicillin.

• In TSS there is ARDS and renal failure due to elaboration of pyrogenic erythrotoxin. Treatment is with heavy dose of penicillin along with clindamycin 600 mg IV 8 hourly.

PNEUMOCOCCAL INFECTIONS

• Pneumococci cause lobar pneumonia, meningitis, otitis and sinusitis, endocarditis.
• In pneumonia there is fever, rigor, pleuritic chest pain, productive cough, lobar consolidation in chest x-rays; lancet-shaped gram positive diplococci in sputum diagnostic. Uncomplicated pneumonia is treated with amoxycillin 750 mg bid for 7–10 days or azithromycin/ clarithromycin for 5–10 days. More seriously ill need penicillin G, 2 MU IV 4 hourly or IV vancomycin (in penicillin allergy patients).
• Pneumococcal endocarditis needs penicillin G, 24 MU IV daily.
• Penicillin resistant pneumococci need ceftriaxone 1 gm IV daily or fluoroquinolones (levofloxacin, gatifloxacin, moxifloxacin).
• Pneumococcal meningitis best treated empirically with ceftriaxone 4 gm IV plus vancomycin 15 mg/kg IV tid till availability of culture sensitivity when penicillin 24 MU daily or ceftriaxone 4 gm daily or chloramphenicol 6 gm daily can be substituted.

STAPHYLOCOCCAL INFECTIONS

• Folliculitis with tendency to abscess formation.
• Osteomyelitis, toxic shock syndrome.
• Gram positive cocci in clusters in staining.
• Mild skin infection is treated with cloxacillin 500 mg or cephalexin 500 mg or erythromycin 500 qid PO. In

severe or extensive infection cefazolin 1 gm IV 8 hrly or vancomycin 1 gm IV bid can be given so also nafcillin 1.5 gm IV 6 hourly.

- For staphylococcal osteomyelitis based on bonescan or gallium scan oxacillin 9–12 gm/day in 6 divided doses or vancomycin for penicillin resistant cases for duration of 4–6 weeks be given.
- In toxic shock syndrome (adults) and scalded skin syndrome (children) important aspects of treatment include rehydration, antistaphylococcal drugs and management of renal or cardiac failure along with drainage of abscess.
- Coagulase negative staphylococci cause infection of intra vascular and prosthetic devices and wound infection following cardiothoracic surgery. Infection is less virulent but more indolent. They need vancomycin 1 gm IV bid or a combination of vancomycin plus rifampicin 300 mg twice daily plus gentamicin 1 mg/kg IV 8 hrly.

GAS GANGRENE (CLOSTRIDIAL MYONECROSIS)

Essentials of diagnosis

- Sudden onset of pain and edema in an area of wound contamination.
- Systemic toxicity, brown to blood tinged watery exudate from wound, skin discolouration around the wound.
- Crepitus around wound, gas seen in x-ray.

Treatment

- Penicillin G, 2 MU, 3 hourly IV along with metronidazole; alternatives are clindamycin, cefoxitin.
- Surgical debridement.
- Hyperbaric oxygen therapy.

TETANUS

Essentials of diagnosis

- Trismus followed by stiffness of neck and other muscles, dysphagia, hyperreflexia and irritability.
- Painful convulsion precipitated by minimum stimuli (opisthotonos).
- Clear consciousness, muscle spasm persisting between convulsions.

Treatment

- Isolation in dark quiet room.
- Tetanus immunoglobulin 5,000 units IM.
- Penicillin 20 MU daily.
- Control of spasm with diazepam, chlorpromazine; in severe cases curare like agents with mechanical ventilation.
- Once patient has recovered, tetanus immunisation with toxoid.

BOTULISM

- Sudden onset of diplopia, dysphagia, dysphonia, dry mouth and muscle weakness progressing to respiratory palsy.
- Pupil dilated and fixed in most cases.
- History of ingestion of tinned, smoked food.
- Clear sensorium and normal body temperature.
- Botulinum antitoxin 20,000 IU be given IM on suspicion of botulism; respiratory palsy needs respiratory support.

ANTHRAX

- Cutaneous anthrax presents as an erythematous papule that becomes vesicular with a black center (eschar) with regional lymphadenopathy.

- Pulmonary anthrax manifests with cough, dyspnoea, sore throat and x-ray evidence of pneumonitis and mediastinitis.
- Smear of skin lesion or sputum shows gram positive encapsulated rods.
- *Treatment* of cutaneous infection is with tetracycline 500 mg qid and pulmonary disease is with penicillin G, 2 MU IV, 4 hrly.

DIPHTHERIA

- Fever, sore throat, nasal discharge, hoarseness, cervical adenopathy (bull neck).
- Tenacious gray membrane in throat, nose or larynx.
- Complicated by myocarditis and cranial neuropathy.
- Immediate administration of 20,000–100,000 units of ADS is life shaving along with erythromycin 500 mg qid for 14 days.
- Active immunisation during childhood is necessary.

LISTERIOSIS

- Listeria can cause meningitis in neonates and immunocompromised adults.
- Neonatal infection acquired in utero (granulomatosis infanti-septicum) presents with disseminated abscess and granuloma.
- Drug of choice is ampicillin 8–12 gm IV daily in 4–6 divided doses combined with gentamicin for first few days; alternatively TMP-SMX for 2–3 weeks (3–6 weeks for meningitis).

WHOOPING COUGH

- Adults act as reservoirs and infants are the sufferers.
- 2 week prodrome of cough, coryza, anorexia followed by paroxysmal cough ending in a high-pitched inspiratory "whoop".

' Absolute lymphocytosis.
' *Treatment* is with azithromycin 500 mg OD or Clarithromycin 500 mg bd or erythromycin 500 mg qid for 10 days.
• Active immunization in childhood and erythromycin prophylaxis to contacts.

LEGIONNAIRE'S DISEASE

• Patients are often immunocompromised, smoker or have chronic lung disease.
• Pleuritic chest pain, toxic appearance, scant sputum.
• Focal patchy infiltrates or consolidation in chest x-ray.
• Sputum Gram stain shows PMN leucocytes but no organism.
• *Treatment* is with erythromycin 1 gm IV 6 hrly followed by 500 mg PO 4 times daily for 14–21 days. Alternatives are azithromycin, clarithromycin, levofloxacin, etc.
• Macrolide + rifampicin or macrolide + fluoroquinolone are reserved for immunocompromised.

GRAM NEGATIVE BACTEREMIA

• Fever and chills of abrupt onset.
• Hyperventilation with respiratory alkalosis are early features.
• Confusion, hypotension and shock.
• Immature forms of PMN leukocytosis, thrombocyto- penia, often DIC.
• *Treatment* is with fluid therapy and pressure agents; (2) treatment of sepsis with appropriate antibiotic, i.e. ticarcilin – clavulanate, imipenem, third generation cephalosporin; (3) anti endotoxin monoclonal antibodies, anti TNF monoclonal antibody or soluble protein C are not helpful; (4) control of DIC, with fresh frozen plasma and heparin.

ENTERIC FEVER

- Gradual onset of sore throat, cough, diarrhoea/constipation.
- Rose spots, relative bradycardia, splenomegaly, abdominal pain and distension.
- Step rising pattern of fever.
- Leucopenia; blood, urine and stool culture positive for salmonella.
- *Complications* include intestinal haemorrhage and perforation, pneumonia, myocarditis, encephalopathy, nephropathy, cholecystitis, osteomyelitis and psychosis.
- *Treatment* is with ciprofloxacin 750 mg bid or ceftriaxone 2 gm daily for 5–10 days. Amoxycillin, sparfloxacin, ofloxacin are equally effective so also chloramphenicol.
- Prevention is by multiple dose oral vaccine or single dose parenteral vaccine.

SHIGELLOSIS

- Diarrhoea with blood and mucus, small quantity, tenesmus.
- Crampy abdominal pain and systemic toxicity.
- White blood cells and RBC in stool; organism isolated on stool culture.
- *Treatment* is by rehydration and prevention of hypotension and renal failure; cipofloxacin 750 mg bid; TMP-SMX Ds 1 bid for 3 days.

CHOLERA

- Voluminous diarrhoea; stool is liquid, gray, turbid and without fecal odor, blood or pus (rice water stool).
- Rapid development of marked dehydration.
- Positive stool culture.
- *Treatment* is replacement of fluids by Ringer lactate and normal saline along with fluoroquinolones,

tetracycline, ampicillin. In mild illness oral rehydration with antibiotic is sufficient.

BRUCELLOSIS

- Insidious onset of intermittent often, undulant chronic fever, arthralgia, headache, sweating, anorexia, weight loss, epididymitis in 10%.
- Hepatosplenomegaly, cervical and axillary lymphadenopathy.
- Lymphocytosis, positive blood culture, elevated agglutination titre.
- *Treatment* is with doxycycline 100 mg bid plus rifampicin 600 mg OD plus streptomycin 1 gm OD for 21 days. Longer duration of therapy is needed for meningitis, osteomyelitis and relapse cases.

TULAREMIA

- Fever, headache, prostration.
- Papule progressing to ulcer at site of inoculation with enlarged regional lymphnodes.
- Culture of ulcer or lymphnode aspirate positive for pasteurella.
- *Treatment* is with streptomycin 0.5 gm IM bid plus tetracycline 500 mg qid or chloramphenicol 500 mg qid.

PLAGUE

- Sudden onset of high fever, muscular pains and prostration. .
- Axillary or inguinal lymphadenopathy (bubo).
- Pneumonitis with cough, tachypnea, blood tinged sputum.
- Bacteremia may supervene with toxic appearance, delirium and coma, purpuric spots (black plague).
- *Treatment* is with streptomycin 1 gm IM stat followed by 0.5 gm IM tid plus tetracycline 500 mg qid .

- Exposed person to risk of plague should receive tetracycline 500 mg bid for 5 days.

CHANCROID

- Causative agent is *Haemophilus ducrey.*
- A vesicopustule turning to painful ulcer with undermined edge and necrotic base on penis or cervix.
- Tender, matted inguinal nodes with overlying erythema, fever, chills and malaise may then develop.
- Balanitis and phimosis may occur.
- Treatment is with azithromycin 1 gm orally or injection ceftriaxone 250 IM once; alternately ciproflaxacin 500 mg bid for 3 days.

GRANULOMA INGUINALE

- Causative agent is *Donovania granulomatis.*
- Insidious onset of painless infiltrated nodules in perineum or genitalia that slough to form shallow sharply demarcated ulcer with beefy red friable base.
- The ulcer heals at one end, the other end advancing with rolled edge of granulation tissue, often advancing to lower abdomen and thigh.
- *Treatment* is with erythromycin 500 mg 4 times daily for 21 days.

BACILLARY ANGIOMATOSIS

- Causative agent is *B. henselae* or *B.quintana.*
- Raised reddish, highly vascular skin lesions mimicking Kaposi's sarcoma but with fever in immuno-compromised.
- Lymphadenopathy, hepatomegaly and osteomyelitis may occur.
- *Treatment* is with doxycycline 100 mg bid or erythromycin 250 mg qid for 14 days but with visceral involvement treatment be continued for months.

- *B. quintana* can also cause trench fever and culture negative endocarditis.

ANAEROBIC INFECTIONS

- Can cause chronic sinusitis, chronic otitis media, mastoiditis, peritonsillar abscess – responding to oral or IV penicillin or clindamycin 300 mg qid or 600 mg IV tid for 7–10 days.
- Can cause necrotising pneumonia (aspiration pneumonia) with foul smelling sputum. Treatment is with clindamycin 300 mg 6 hrly or penicillin 2 MU IV 4 hrly to be followed by amoxycillin 500 mg qid to complete therapy duration of 3–4 weeks.
- Can cause brain abscess, subdural empyema, CNS thrombophlebitis. Treatment is penicillin 20 MU, IV daily along with metronidazole 750 mg IV tid for 6–8 weeks. Former two require drainage.
- Can cause intra-abdominal abscess — appendicular abscess, perirectal abscess, diverticulitis. Treatment is IV metronidazole with imipenem or ampicillin – sulbactam for severe disease. Clindamycin, cefotetan and cefoxitin are also effective. Mild disease can be treated with ciprofloxacin 750 mg bid with metronidazole 500 mg tid.
- Endocarditis by anaerobes be treated with penicillin 12–20 million units IV daily for 4–6 weeks.
- Skin and soft tissue infection like bacterial synergistic gangrene, necrotising fascitis, nonclostridial crepitant cellulitis needs broad spectrum antibiotic for anaerobes and other bacteria i.e. vancomycin plus metronidazole plus gentamicin/tobramycin for 15 days.

ACTINOMYCOSIS

- Causative agent *Actinomyces israeli.*
- Cervicofacial actinomycosis: Indurated mass, usually painless, progressing to abscess formation and

discharge of sulfur granules. There may be bone involvement.

- Abdominal actinomycosis: Irregular ileocecal mass with spiking fever and chills, vomiting, weight loss.
- Thoracic actinomycosis Fever, night sweat, pleuritic pain, weight loss, productive cough, multiple sinuses in chest wall.
- All forms treated by penicillin 10–20 million units IV daily followed by penicillin V 500 mg qid for weeks to months, often combined with surgical drainage and resection.
- Actinomycetoma that has deep invasion, bone destruction with multiple abscess on skin is treated with dapsone 100 mg daily/TMP SMX combined with streptomycin up to 1 gm IM daily.

NOCARDIOSIS

- Causative agent *Nocardia asteroides*, common to immunocompromised.
- Pulmonary involvement causes night sweats, weight loss, fever, purulent sputum. X-ray shows infiltration.
- Dissemination to other organs may occur.
- *Treatment* is with IV TMP-SMX followed by oral therapy continued for at least 6 months.

ORNITHOSIS

- Causative agent *Chlamydia psittaci.*
- Rapid onset of fever, chill, dry cough, with X-ray evidence of atypical pneumonia (interstitial and diffuse).
- *Treatment* is with tetracyline 0.5 mg IV bid or 500 mg PO qid for 14–21 days. Erythromycin is also effective.
- *Chlamydia pneumoniae* also causes atypical pneumonia and probably plays a role in coronary atherosclerosis; treatment is as for ornithosis. Levofloxacin 500 mg OD in addition is also effective.

SYPHILIS

- Causative agent is *Treponema pallidum.*
- Primary syphilis: Painless genital ulcer with clean indurated base and firm indurated border (button ulcer); can occur on lips, perianal area, rectum; nontender lymphadenopathy.
- Secondary syphilis: Maculopapular nonitchy rash, diffuse, involving palm and sole; painless silvery ulcerations of mucous membrane with surrounding erythema; condyloma lata; constitutional symptoms (fever, malaise, arthralgia), iridocyclitis, hepatitis, meningitis, cranial neuropathy (II-III) and glomerulonephritis.
- Neurosyphilis: (a) Meningovascular presenting as hemiplegia, seizure (b) Tabes dorsalis with impaired proprioception and vibration, Argyll Robertson pupil, ataxia, cranial neuropathy (II-VIII), Charcot joint (c) general paresis – decreased memory, optic atrophy, personality changes, hyperactive reflexes.
- Cardiovascular syphilis: Aortic aneurysm, coronary osteal stenosis and aortic insufficiency.
- Gumma involving skin, mucous membrane and bone. The last three constitute late (tertiary) syphilis.
- FTA-ABS is most dependable test for diagnosis.
- *Treatment* of primary syphilis is with benzathine penicillin 2.4 MU IM once. Alternatively doxycycline 100 mg bid or tetracycline 500 mg qid for 2 weeks can be given.
- *Treatment* of secondary syphilis is as for primary disease unless ocular disease or CNS involvement is present, in which case treatment is as for neurosyphilis.
- *Treatment* of cardiovascular syphilis is with benzathine penicillin 2.4 MU weekly for 3 doses, else tetracycline or doxcline be given for 28 days.
- Neurosyphilis is treated with procaine penicillin 2.4 MU IM daily with 500 mg probenecid PO qid for 10–14 days

or Penicillin 18–24 MU daily IV in 6 divided doses for 14 days.

• In late syphilis serologic tests remain positive despite treatment. In neurosyphilis benzathine penicillin 2.4 MU weekly for 3 doses should follow 14 days of procaine/ penicillin G. CSF be examined at 6 month interval and if cell count is still abnormal another course of procaine penicillin be given.

NONSEXUALLY TRANSMITTED TREPONEMATOSIS

• *Yaws* is granulomatous lesion of skin, bone and mucous membrane. Mother yaws is a painless papule that later ulcerates with painless lymphadenopathy. Secondary lesions appear 6–12 weeks later. Bone involvement causes shortening of digits. Benzathine penicillin 2.4 million units is curative.

• *Pinta* caused by *T. carateum* is non ulcerating spreading papulosquamous plaque showing colour changes followed by secondary lesions. Penicillin in doses as above is treatment of choice.

RELAPSING FEVER

• Caused by *Borrelia* species, can be of epidemic or endemic type.

• Fever, chill, headache, arthralgia of abrupt onset with hepatosplenomegaly, psychic and neurologic symptoms. Attack terminates abruptly only to return repeatedly after 7–10 days. Treatment is with single dose of procaine penicillin. In endemic form 5–10 days of therapy is adequate.

RATBITE FEVER

• Causative agent is *Spirillum minus.*

- Rat bite site becomes swollen, indurated and painful with regional lymphadenitis, fever, arthralgia continuing for 3–4 days followed by remission and repeated relapse. *Treatment* is with procaine penicillin 6 lac units IM bid for 10–14 days or tetracycline 0.5 gm every 6 hour for 10–14 days.

LEPTOSPIROSIS

- *L. haemorrhagica* causes most severe illness with initial septicemic phase of abrupt fever, chills, headache, and myalgia to be followed by jaundice, bleeding, mental obtundation, hypotension and even death. In other forms of leptospirosis the septicemic phase remits followed by immune phase when leptospira disappear with recurrence of symptoms and with meningitis, uveitis, etc. but complete recovery. Doxycycline 100 mg bid for 7 days or penicillin 6 MU daily IV for 7 days are effective. Doxycycline 200 mg orally weekly provides effective prophylaxis.

LYME DISEASE

- Causative spirochete is *Borrelia burgdorferi.*
- Disease evolves in 3 phases. (1) Early localised infection with erythema migrans and flu-like illness, (2) Early dissemination phase with skin lesions, aseptic meningitis, Bell's palsy, encephalopathy, musculo-skeletal symptoms. (3) Late persistent phase with large joint arthritis, subacute encephalopathy and acrodermatitis chronicum atrophicans.
- *Treatment* is with doxycycline 100 mg bid or amoxycillin 500 mg tid or cefuroxine 500 mg twice daily – all for 3–4 weeks. In CNS involvement ceftriaxon 2 gm IV once daily or penicillin 18–24 millions IV daily for 2–4 weeks. Chronic Lyme disease or post Lyme disease syndrome only needs symptomatic treatment.

LEISHMANIASIS

- Can be of 3 forms (1) Visceral leishmaniasis, known as kala azar caused by *L. donovani* (2) Cutaneous leishmaniasis caused by *L. tropica* (3) Mucocutaneous leishmaniasis known as espundia caused by *L. braziliensis* and (4) diffuse cutaneous leishmaniasis.
- In kala azar there is fever with hepatosplenomegaly and anaemia; weight loss, pigmentation of skin of face.
- Post kala azar dermal leishmaniasis is characterised by multiple nodules, butterfly erythema and hypopigmented macules.
- In espundia cutaneous ulcerative lesion is followed by destructive nasopharyngeal lesions.
- In diffuse cutaneous leishmaniasis there is leprosy like skin lesions.
- Discovery of intracellular nonflagellated amastigotes in bone marrow, skin, liver and spleen are diagnostic.
- *Treatment* is with: (1) Sodium stibogluconate 20 mg/kg/d for 20 days in cutaneous leishmaniasis and 28 days for visceral and mucocutaneous leishmaniasis. Treatment be discontinued if there is hepatic damage or myocarditis. (2) Pentamidine isetheonate 2–4 mg/kg IM daily or alt-day, 14 doses for visceral and 4 doses for cutaneous leishmaniasis. (3) Amphotericin B 1 mg/kg daily IV for 20 days or liposomal amphotericin 3 mg/kg/d on days 1–5, 14 and 21 are effective in visceral leishmaniasis. (4) Paromomycin 15% topical application is effective in cutaneous disease or IV in visceral leishmaniasis.

TRYPANOSOMIASIS

- Can be of African form (sleeping sickness) caused by *T. rhodesiense* or American form (Chaga's disease) caused by *T. cruzi.*
- In sleeping sickness there is early haemolymphatic stage with irregular fever, papular skin rash,

generalised lymphadenopathy, hepatosplenomegaly and anaemia followed by a meningoencephalitic phase of somnolence, speech and gait disorder, tremor etc.

- In Chaga's disease there is inflammatory lesion at the site of inoculation with prolonged fever, hepatosplenomegaly, lymphadenopathy and myocarditis followed by a chronic phase characterised by cardiac arrhythmias, heart failure, megaesophagus and megacolon, conduction disturbances and thrombo embolism.
- Diagnosis is based on recovery of motile organism in blood, bone marrow or CSF.
- *Treatment* of sleeping sickness is with suramin 1 gm on days 1, 3, 7, 14, 21 or pentamidine 4 mg/kg/d IM for 10 days.
- With CNS involvement, since above drugs do not cross blood brain barrier treatment is with IV eflornithine 400 mg/kg/d in 4 divided doses for 14 days.
- Treatment of Chaga's disease is only under taken at acute phase with nifurtimox 8–10 mg/kg/d PO in 4 divided dose for 3–4 months or benznidazole. Drugs are not of much use in chronic phase.

AMOEBIASIS

- *E. histolytica* can cause mild to moderate colitis, severe colitis, and hepatic disease.
- Colitis is characterised by recurrent diarrhoea, abdominal cramp, mucous in stool. In severe colitis blood in stool, fever, ileus, perforation can occur. Colon is thick and tender in chronic disease.
- In hepatic amoebiasis there is tender hepatomegaly, fever, chill and leukocytosis. US is diagnostic.
- Localised granulomatous lesions of the colon (amoeboma) can present as annular constricting mass or irregular lesion projecting into bowel with pain and obstructing symptoms to simulate in X-ray as malignancy and tuberculosis.

- Diagnosis is based on discovery of trophozoites in liquid stool and cysts in formed stool. Indirect haemagglutination test is insensitive in early infection and does not distinguish recent form past infection.
- *Treatment* of mild to moderate colitis is with metronidazole 750 mg tid for 10 days or tinidazole 800 mg tid for 3 days, combined with diloxanide furoate 500 mg tid for 10 days or dihydroxyquin 650 mg tid for 21 days. In severe colitis emetine or dehydroemetine 1 mg/kg SC (mxm daily dose of emetine is 65 mg and dehydroemetine 90 mg) for 3–5 days followed by tetracycline 250 mg qid for 10 days along with diloxanide furoate to be followed by chloroquine 300 mg base twice daily for 2 days and 150 mg base bid for 19 days.
- Hepatic amoebiasis can be treated by metronidazole/tinidazole plus diloxanide furoate/iodoquinol followed by chloroquine or with the drugs outlined for severe colitis.

Table 1.1: Differentiation between amoebic and bacillary dysentery

Features	Amoebic dysentery	Bacillary dysentery
Number of stools per day	6 to 8 motions per day	More than 10 motions per day
Amount	Relatively copious	Small quantity
Odour	Offensive	Odourless
Colour	Dark red	Bright red
Nature	Blood and mucus mixed with faeces	Blood and mucus (with minimal fecal matter
Reacion	Acid	Alkaline
Consistency	Not adherent to the container	Adherent to the container
Microscopic Examination		
a) RBC	In clumps	Discrete
b) Pus cells	Scanty	Numerous
c) Eosinophils	Present	Absent
e) Parasite	Trophozoites of *E. histolytica*	Nil

AMOEBIC MENINGOENCEPHALITIS

- Caused by *Naegleria flowlere* with fulminating haemorrhagic necrotising meningoencephalitis which is rapidly fatal.
- CSF shows leukocytosis and amoebas can be recovered from it.
- *Treatment* is with amphotericin B plus rifampicin.
- Acanthamoeba cause granulomatous multifocal chronic necrotising encephalitis, skin lesions resembling deep fungal infection and keratitis. *Treatment* is with ketoconazole, amphotericin, itraconazole, pentamidine, fluocytosine, etc. but mostly ineffective. Keratitis may respond to topical propamidine isethionate (0.1%), polyhexamethylene biguanide, chlorhexidine digluconate and oral itraconazole.

BABESIOSIS

- Causative agent is *Babesia microti*, often coinfecting with Lyme disease and ehrlichiosis; most severe in immunosuppressed.
- The illness is characterised by irregular fever, chills, headache, diaphoresis and often with hepatosplenomegaly, haemoglobinuria, haemolytic anaemia and thrombocytopenia.
- Diagnosis is based on discovery of parasite within RBC.
- *Treatment* is with quinine 650 mg tid for 7 days plus clindamycin 650 mg tid or azithromycin 500 mg bid for 7 days plus atovaquone 750 mg twice daily for 7 days.

BALANTIDIASIS

- Causative agent is *B. coli*, a large ciliated intestinal protozoa.

- Causes chronic recurrent diarrhoea alternating with constipation but bloody diarrhoea with tenesmus can occur.
- *Treatment* of choice is tetracycline 500 mg qid for 10 days or iodoquinol 650 mg tid x 21 days.

CRYPTOSPORIDIOSIS

- Coccidiosis and microsporidiosis are intracellular infections of intestinal epithelial cells by spore forming protozoa.
- Cryptospora cause diarrhoea in immunocompetent and microspora cause diarrhoea in HIV patients.
- Biliary infection can occur in all of them with sclerosing cholangitis and acalculous cholecystitis. Microsporidia also cause corneal disease.
- Intestinal infection is nonulcerative and noninvasive with diarrhoea, cramping, malabsorption, weightloss, and mucous in stool.
- TMP-SMX (DS) 4 times daily for 10 days, then twice daily for 3 weeks is effective in isosporiasis and cyclosporiasis. Albendazole 400 mg tid x 3 months is effective in microsporidiosis but no treatment is available for sacrocytosis and cryptosporidiosis. However, roxithromycin 300 mg twice daily for 4 weeks, spiramycin 1 gm tid for 2 weeks, AZT, eflornithine, letrazuril may be tried.

GIARDIASIS

- Causative agent is *Giardia lamblia* causing acute or chronic diarrhoea and malabsorption. Abdominal distention, belching, flatulence, cramps after meals are common. Diagnosed from presence of cysts/trophozoites in feces or duodenal aspirate.
- *Treatment* is with metronidazole 250 mg tid for 3–7 days or tinidazole 2 gm single dose/secnidazole/ornidazole or furazolidine 100 mg tid for 7 days.

SCHISTOSOMIASIS

• Caused by *S. haematobium, S. japonicum* and *S. mansoni*.
• In acute phase (Katayama fever) there is diarrhoea, myalgia, dry cough, fever, hepatomegaly and eosinophilia.
• In chronic phase there is terminal haematuria, bladder calcification, urinary frequency (*S. haematobium*) or hepatosplenomegaly, bleeding from esophageal varices (*S. mansoni, S. japonicum*), often with pulmonary hypertension and heart failure.
• Diagnosis is based on discovery of eggs in urine or stool.
• *Treatment* is with praziquantel 20 mg/kg twice a day for 1 day in *S. haematobium* and *S. mansoni* and thrice a day for one day for *S. japonicum*. Oxamniquine 15 mg/kg once is effective for *S.mansoni*.

FASCIOLOPSIASIS

• Causative fluke is *F. buski*, causing intestinal infection with abdominal pain and diarrhoea. Heavy infection can cause intestinal obstruction, cachexia. Praziquantel 25 mg/kg tid for a day is curative. Alternative drug is niclosamide.

FASCIOLIASIS

• *F. hepatica* inhabits biliary and hepatic system and causes (a) acute symptoms like tender hepatomegaly, high fever, leukocytosis and marked eosinophilia; (b) chronic obstructive symptoms — sclerosing cholangitis, choledocholithiasis and biliary cirrhosis. Praziquantel 25 mg/kg tid for 7 days may be effective, else emetine/dehydroemetine is worth trying.

PARAGONIMIASIS

• *P. westeremani* is a lung fluke causing dry cough and low-grade fever initially progressing to pleuritic pain, rusty sputum, often complicated by bronchiectasis, pulmonary fibrosis and pleural thickening. Chest x-ray may show infiltrates, fibrosis, nodules, cavitary lesion, pleural thickening and calcification. Cerebral disease manifests with seizure, cranial neuropathy and CT scan shows multilocular ring lesions.

- *Treatment* is with praziquantel 25 mg/kg tid for 30 days. Alternative drug is bithionol 30–50 mg/kg on alternative day for 10–15 doses.

TAPEWORM INFECTIONS

- Beef tape worm is by *T. saginata*; pork tapeworm is by *T. solium*, fish tape worm is by *D. latum*, dwarf tapeworm is by *H.nana*, rodent tape worm is by *H. diminuta* and dog tapeworm is by *D. caninum*. Symptoms are often vague with abdominal pain, diarrhoea, hunger, etc. Fish tapeworm causes Vitamin B_{12} deficiency with pernicious anaemia. Eggs can be seen in stool.
- Praziquantel 10 mg/kg single dose is curative for *T. solium* and *T. saginata*. Niclosamide 2 gm single dose is equally effective. For *H. nana* praziquantel 25 mg/kg is also effective.

CYSTICERCOSIS

- History of exposure to *T. solium*, concomitant or past intestinal infection.
- Seizure and other symptoms and signs of focal space occupying lesion.
- Subcutaneous or muscular nodules, calcified lesions on x-rays of soft tissues.
- Calcified or uncalcified cyst in CT scan/MRI, positive serological tests.
- Brain cysts can be parenchymal, ventricular, in subarachnoid space and meninges and in spinal cord, can also assume form of grape like irregular clusters; can be seen as free floating in vitreous causing scotoma.

- Albendazole and praziquantel are both effective. Albendazole 15 mg/kg in two divided doses with fatty meal for 8–28 days or praziquantel 50–100 mg/kg/d in 3 divided doses for 10–30 days with fatty meal are usually sufficient combined with prednisolone 30 mg/day with gradual tapering over 2 weeks; seizure control with antiepileptics be continued for few months. Intraventricular, racemose and subarachnoid cysts respond less; calcified cysts need no treatment.

ECHINOCOCCOSIS

- Causative agent *E. granulosus* or *E. multilocularis*.
- Can encyst in liver, lung, brain and mediastinum to produce symptoms by pressure, leak or rupture.
- Hepatic cysts can present with right upper quadrant pain, biliary obstruction, secondary cholangitis, cirrhosis and portal hypertension.
- Pulmonary cyst can obstruct bronchus with lung collapse.
- Brain cysts cause seizure and raised ICT. Bone cysts can erode bone with pain and spontaneous fracture.
- Vertebral cysts can cause paraplegia.
- *Treatment* is with albendazole 800 mg daily for 3 months, if cyst does not disappear surgical removal is warranted. Percutaneous aspiration and injection of scolicidal agent can be undertaken under US guidance. Prazinquantel has a supportive role.
- *E. multilocularis* cyst in liver behaves like a neoplasm that infiltrates and proliferates requiring surgical removal of entire larval mass.

ANISAKIASIS

- Causative agents are larvae of anisakid nematodes that fail to mature. In acute form presentation may mimic surgical abdomen with mild fever, diarrhoea, pain abdomen, diffuse abdominal tenderness. In chronic form symptoms may mimic gastric ulcer, gastritis, gastric tumor, bowel obstruction and inflammatory bowel disease.

- In acute disease larvae can be seen in gastroscopy and in chronic disease small bowel x-ray may show thickening and segmental stenosis.
- There is no specific drug treatment, except for symptomatic treatment.

ANGIOSTRONGYLIASIS

- Causative larvae are of *A. cantonensis* and *A. costarinensis.*
- Usual clinical findings in *A. cantonensis* are those of meningoencephalitis, asymmetric transient cranial neuropathies. CSF shows eosinophilic pleocytosis.
- No specific drug is available but albendazole 400 mg bid for 7 days, mebendazole 100 mg bid for 5 days, thiaebendazole 25 mg/kg tid for 3 days may be tried.
- *A. costarinensis* larvae mature in mesenteric vessels causing vasculitis and bowel ischaemia, perforation, bleeding, infarction. No specific therapy is available but albendazole, thiabendazole, etc. can be tried.

ASCARIASIS

- Causative agent *A. lumbricoides.*
- In pulmonary phase there is transient cough, wheezing, urticaria and transient pulmonary infiltrates.
- In intestinal phase vague abdominal pain and often intestinal obstruction or bile duct obstruction.
- Eggs can be discovered in stool.
- *Treatment* is with albendazole 400 mg single dose, pyrantel palmoate 10 mg/kg single dose, piperazine 75 mg/kg (mxm 3.5 g) for 2 days or levamisole 150 mg single dose.

CREEPING ERUPTION

- Caused by migrating larvae of *A. caninum.*
- Pruritic erythematous papules at site of larval entry followed by advancing serpiginous erruption.
- *Treatment* is with ivermectin 200 g/kg single dose or albendazole 400 mg bid for 5 days.

DRACUNCULIASIS

- Causative agent is *D. medinensis* causing skin blister with erythema, burning, tenderness and ulceration. Ankle and knee joint infections with resultant deformity are common complications.
- *Treatment* is manual extraction but drugs like metronidazole 250 mg tid for 10 days, mebendazole, thiabendazole that alleviate symptoms but do not kill the worms be tried.

ENTEROBIASIS

- Causative agent is *E. vermicularis* causing nocturnal perianal and vulvar pruritus and irritability, vague gastrointestinal symptoms. Worm migration can cause vulvovaginitis, appendicitis, diverticulitis, cystitis, granulomatous reactions of colon.
- *Treatment* is with albendazole 400 mg, mebendazole 100 mg or pyrantel palmoate 10 mg/kg, all repeated at 2 and 4 weeks.

GNATHOSTOMIASIS

- Causative agent is *G. spinigerum* whose larvae migrate to cause epigastric pain, urticaria, eosinophilia, prutritic subcutaneous swellings and invasion of internal organs with haematemesis, haemoptysis, spontaneous pneumothorax, eosinophilic meningoencephalitis, etc.
- *Treatment* is with albendazole 400 mg bid for 21 days.

ANKYLOSTOMIASIS

- Causative agents: *A. duodenale* and *Nectar americanus.*
- Clinical manifestations include pruritic erythematous dermatitis at site of larval entry; dry cough, wheezing, blood tinged sputum during pulmonary migration and iron deficiency anaemia, hypoproteinemia, abdominal pain and peptic ulcer like symptoms due to adult worms in intestine.
- *Treatment* is with albendazole 400 mg once, mebendazole 100 mg bd for 3 days, pyrantel palmoate 10 mg/kg once.

STRONGYLOIDIASIS

- Causative agent is *S. stercoralis.*
- Pruritic dermatitis at site of larval penetration, diarrhoea, epigastric pain, cough transient pulmonary infiltrates, eosinophilia.
- Severe diarrhoea, bronchopneumonia, ileus, pleuro-pericarditis, cholecystitis in hyperinfection syndrome.
- *Treatment* is with ivermectin 200 µg/kg for 2 days or thiabendazole 25 mg/kg twice daily for 2–3 days, repeated after 2 weeks.

TRICHINOSIS

- Causative agent – *T. spiralis.*
- First week – diarrhoea, cramps, malaise.
- Second week onwards – muscle pain and tenderness, fever, facial and periorbital edema, conjunctivitis, photo-phobia.
- Eosinophilia, larvae in muscle biopsy.
- *Treatment* is with albendazole 400 mg bid for 10 days in intestinal phase; mebendazole and thiabendazole are the alternatives.
- In muscle invasion stage corticosteroids for 1–2 days followed by long term low dose maintenance combined with albendazole.

TRICHURIASIS

* Caused by *T. trichura*; light infection is asymptomatic, in heavy infection abdominal cramps, tenesmus, diarrhoea, distention, flatulence, rectal prolapse may occur.
* *Treatment* is with albendazole 400 mg single dose, mebendazole 100 mg bid or oxantel palmoate 10–15 mg/kg for 2–5 days.

TOXOCARIASIS

* Caused by *T. canis*; as the hatched larvae fail to mature they migrate (visceral larva migrans) to lodge in various organs and cause cough, fever, wheezing, hepatosplenomegaly and lymphadenopathy, carditis, encephalomyelitis, etc. with marked leukocytosis.
* In ocular toxocariasis, there is impairment of vision, squint, red eye due to eosinophilic granuloma of retina that resembles retinoblastoma requiring CT scan of orbit for diagnosis.
* For acute infection mebendazole 100 mg bid for 21 days, albendazole 400 mg bid for 21 days and diethyl carbamazine 6 mg/kg for 21 days may be given along with antibiotic, corticosteroids and antihistaminics.
* Ocular toxoplasmosis is treated with oral and subconjunctival steroid, anthelmintics as above, vitrectomy and photocoagulation.

FILARIASIS

* Causative agent *W. bancrofti* and *B. malayi*.
* Fever, lymphangitis at irregular intervals often involving testis and epididymis (epididymo orchitis), pelvic, abdominal and retroperitoneal lymphatics.
* In chronic phase lymphatic obstruction leads to hydrocele, scrotal lymphedema, elephantiasis of vulva,

legs, breast; chyluria may occur due to rupture of bladder lymphatics.

- In tropical pulmonary eosinophilia there is episodic nocturnal coughing and wheezing, dyspnoea, low grade fever, scant expectoration, obstructive-restrictive defect in PFT with eosinophilia and high filarial antibody titre and IgE levels.
- In acute stage *treatment* is with antistreptococcal antibiotics (secondary invaders) along with diethylcarbamazine 2 mg/kg tid for 21 days. Ivermectin 200 µg/kg single dose repeated at 6 months kills microfilariae but not adult worms unlike DEC. Albendazole-ivermectin combination is a better microfilaricide.

LOIASIS

- Caused by *Loa loa* producing limb edema or Calabar swellings. The latter are subcutaneous edematous reactions, nonpitting and nonerythematous, with low grade fever and pruritus appearing off and on. Treatment is with DEC starting with 50 mg OD day 1, 50 mg tid day 2, 100 mg tid day 3–21 days.

ONCHOCERCIASIS

- Caused by *Onchocerca vulvulus*, the adult worms living in fibrous subcutaneous nodules releasing microfilariae into skin, lymphatics and eyes. Pruritus, pigmentary skin changes, lymphadenopathy, blindness due to chorioretinitis, optic neuritis, iritis, sclerosing keratitis, glaucoma, cataract, etc. are known.
- Microfilarae can be seen in skin snips, in cornea and anterior chamber.
- *Treatment* is with ivermectin 150 µg/kg in empty stomach with fasting for 2 more hours. Prednisolone 1 mg/kg/day be given to avoid eye reaction. DEC is

equally effective. Ivermectin be repeated monthly for 3 doses. Non responders may be tried with suràmin or amocarzine.

CANDIDIASIS

- Forms part of normal flora but is also opportunistic pathogen.
- Causes mucosal disease, esophagitis and systemic fungemia, endocarditis.
- Persistent oral or vaginal candidiasis should arouse suspicion of HIV infection.
- Esophagitis causes substernal odynophagia, GE reflux and endoscopy with biopsy is confirmatory.
- *Treatment* is with fluconazole 100 mg PO daily or itraconazole solution (10 mg/ml) 100 mg daily for 10–14 days; else amphotericin B 0.3 mg/kg/day IV.
- Vulvovaginal candidiasis causes pruritus, burning, vaginal cheesy discharge and dyspareunia.
- *Treatment* is with 200 mg miconazole vaginal suppository for 3 days or clotrimazole 100 mg vaginal tab for 7 days or fluconazole 150 mg PO.
- Candidal funguria is treated with fluconazole 200 mg daily for 7–14 days or amphotericin B.
- Candidal fungemia with identified retinal lesion need amphotericin IV up total dose of 1 gm; or flucytosine 150 mg/kg/d PO in 4 divided doses is added if CNS involvement occurs. Fluconazole 200–400 mg IV daily is alternative to amphotericin B.
- *Candida krusei* is responsible for over 50% cases of fungemia and is resistant to imidazoles.

HISTOPLASMOSIS

- Caused by *H. capsulatum*; manifests with (1) acute histoplasmosis (fever, x-ray evidence of pneumonia); (2) progressive disseminated histoplasmosis (fever, dyspnoea, hepatosplenomegaly); (3) chronic progressive pulmonary histoplasmosis with apical cavities, mediastinal lymphadenopathy; (4) disseminated disease in immunosuppressed.

- Mild to moderate disease is treated with itraconazole 200–400 mg/d PO and severe disease with amphotericin B.

CRYPTOCOCCOSIS

- Causative agent *C. neoformans*, an encapsulated budding cyst, most common cause of fungal meningitis, obstructive hydrocephalus may occur.
- Oral fluconazole 400 mg PO daily for 10 weeks in moderate disease and amphotericin B IV for 14 days followed by fluconazole for severe disease, e.g. HIV patients be given.

ASPERGILLOSIS

- Caused by *A. fumigatus, A. nijar.*
- Allergic bronchopulmonary aspergillosis manifests with bronchospasm, fleeting pulmonary infiltrates with eosinophilia, high IgE and aspergillus precipitins in blood; can lead to saccular bronchiectasis and fibrotic lung disease; treated with prednisolone 1 mg/kg/d tapered over several months along with itraconazole 200 mg daily for 10 weeks.
- Aspergilloma formation in existing pulmonary cavities causes haemoptysis; treatment is surgical resection.
- Invasive aspergillosis occurs in immunocompromised with severe necrotising pneumonia, ulcerative tracheobronchitis, meningoencephalitis etc.
- *Treatment* of invasive aspergillosis is with amphoterisin B 0.8–1.5 mg/kg/day IV up to total dose of 2 gm, capsofungin 50 mg IV daily may be added. For less severe disease oral itraconazole 200–400 mg/day PO.

MUCORMYCOSIS

* Predisposing conditions include diabetes mellitus, chronic renal failure, steroid/cytotoxic drug use.
* Predilection for nasal sinuses, orbits and lungs and often cerebral invasion.
* *Treatment* is with high dose amphotericin 1–10 mg/kg/day IV.

MADUROMYCOSIS

* Local, slowly progressive destructive infection beginning as papule, nodule and abscess progressing slowly to multiple sinus tracts, deep tissue invasion. Prolonged ketoconazole or itraconazole therapy may help but may ultimately need amputation.

BLASTOMYCOSIS

* Pulmonary infection is common with cough, dyspnoea, chest pain progressing to weight loss, haemoptysis, pleuritic chest pain; x-ray chest shows infiltration with lymphadenopathy.
* Raised verrucous cutaneous lesions with abrupt downward sloping border present in disseminated blastomycosis. Bones may be involved but CNS invasion is rare.
* *Treatment* is with itraconazole 200 mg/day for 2 months, else, amphotericin B.

SPOROTRICHOSIS

* Hard nontender subcutaneous nodule that ulcerates and is followed by similar nodules in the area of lymphatic drainage.
* Disseminated disease may occur in alcoholics and immunocompromised with involvement of lung, bone and CNS.

- *Treatment* is with itraconazole 200–400 mg daily for several months. For localised lymphocutaneous disease potassium iodide orally is an alternative but amphotericin B is reserved for severe disseminated disease.

MALARIA

Essentials of Diagnosis

- Periodic attacks of sequential chills, fever and sweating
- Headache, anaemia, splenomegaly, leukopenia.
- Characteristic parasites in RBC, positive antigen tests
- Complications of falciparum malaria like (1) cerebral (mental disturbances, convulsion, neurologic signs) (2) haemolytic anaemia with jaundice; (3) cholera like stool (algid malaria); (4) ARDS; (5) acute renal failure; (6) hypoglycemia; (7) lactic acidosis; (8) hyperpyrexia; (9) acute hepatopathy with centrilobular necrosis and marked jaundice but no liver failure; (10) adrenal insufficiency with shock; and (11) cardiac dysrhythmia.

Treatment

(1) Treatment of all strains except chloroquine resistant *P. falciparum* is with chloroquine 600 mg base initially, then 300 mg base at 24, 48 hours; for *P. vivax* and *P.ovale* primaquine 15 mg base in addition is given daily for 14 days starting on day 4 and chloroquine 300 mg base can be repeated on day 10 and 17. Patients of *P. falciparum* are given 45 mg of primaquine base single dose after chloroquine to kill gametocytes. If attack is severe quinine or quinidine can be started followed by chloroquine and primaquin or else arteether (see below) can be given.
(2) For chloroquine resistant falciparum strains (1) Quinine 10 mg/kg tid for 3–7 days plus one of the following (a) doxycycline 100 mg bid for 7 days, (b)

clindamycin 900 mg tid for 5 days, (c) pyrimethamine 75 mg + sulfadoxine 1500 mg, (d) tetracycline 500 mg qid for 7 days.

or

Malarone (proguanil 100 mg + atovaquone 250 mg)	2 tab twice daily for 3 days

or

Atovaquone 100 mg + doxycycline 500 mg	twice daily for 3 days

or

Proguanil 100 mg + dapsone 100 mg	twice daily for 3 days

or

Artesunate 4 mg/kg for 3 days followed by mefloquine.

For severe disease

IV quinine/quinidine 10 mg/kg in 5% DW tid followed by oral quinine along with IV doxycycline/clindamycin to complete 7 days of treatment.
or
Artemether 1.6 mg/kg IM twice daily on day 1 and once daily there after for 4 days
or
Arte ether 100 mg IM daily for 3 days
or
Artesunate, 2 mg/kg stat, followed by 1 mg/kg twice daily
or
100 mg PO bid day-1, then 50 mg bid for 4 days.
All artemisinin preparation are to be followed by mefloquine 1250 mg PO.

Prophylactic treatment

(a) In chloroquine sensitive areas — chloroquine 300 mg base weekly, started 1 week before and continued 4 weeks after leaving endemic area

(b) In chloroquine resistant areas – (1) mefloquine 250 mg once weekly, (2) doxycycline 100 mg daily, (3) atovaquone – proguanil 2 tab daily.

2

RENAL DISEASES

ACUTE RENAL FAILURE (ARF)

Essentials of diagnosis

- Oliguria — anuria.
- Nausea, vomiting, altered sensorium due to azotemia often with asterixis, confusion and seizure.
- Platelet dysfunction with bleeding (usually from GI tract), diffuse abdominal pain, ileus.
- Pericarditis often with effusion and cardiac tamponade.
- Raised BUN and creatinine, hyperkalemia, increased anion gap, hyperphosphatemia, hypocalcemia.
- Haematuria, hypertension in glomerulonephritis.
- Serum BUN to creatinine ratio is ≤ 20:1 in ARF due to acute interstitial nephritis and acute tubular necrosis (see Table 2.1).
- Urinary sediments — hyaline casts in prerenal azotemia, pigmented granular and renal tubular casts in ATN, dysmorphic red cells and red cells casts in acute glomerulonephritis; white cells and white cell casts in interstitial nephrosis.

Table 2.1: Urinary indices useful in distinguishing pre-renal from renal causes of oliguria

Indices	Pre-renal	Renal (acute tubular necrosis)
Urine osmolality (mosm/kg)	>500	<350
Urine sodium (mEq/L)	<20	>40
Urine/serum creatinine	>40	<20
Urine/serum osmolality	>1.2	<1.2
Fractional excreted sodium	<1	>1
Renal failure index	<1	>1
Urine specific gravity	>1.020	<1.010

Treatment

- Protein restriction to 0.5 gm/kg/d.
- Furosemide 20–160 mg twice daily PO/IV; or by infusion; else chlorthiazide 500 mg IV 8–12 hours.
- Phosphate binding by oral aluminum hydroxide 500 mg – 1500 mg thrice daily; avoid magnessium salts.
- Calcium supplement.
- Regulation of drug dosage for agents excreted or metabolised by kidneys.
- Prophylactic antibiotics.
- Dialysis if there is hyperkalemia, volume overload unresponsive to diuretics, worsening acidosis and uremic complications (encephalopathy, pericarditis).
- Methylprednisolone 1 gm/day for 1–4 days or oral prednisolone for drug induced interstitial nephritis.
- Plasma exchange is good for Goodpasture's disease.
- Steroids and cytotoxic for immune mediated glomerulonephritis.

CHRONIC RENAL FAILURE (CRF)

Essentials of diagnosis

- Progressive azotemia over months to years.
- Symptoms and signs of uremia (anorexia, nausea, vomiting, fishy odor, hiccup, nocturia, impotence, cramps in legs, anaemia, ecchymoses, pruritus, pleural effusion, hypertension, isosthenuria, peripheral neuropathy).
- Broad casts in urinary sediment.
- Bilateral small kidneys in US (except for amyloidosis, myeloma, diabetic nephropathy) < 10 cm.
- X-ray evidence of renal osteodystrophy, subperiosteal resorption along the radial sides of digits.
- Hyperkalemia occurs when GFR is < 10 ml/min.

Treatment

- Protein restriction to 0.6 gm/kg/day, salt and water restriction to 2 gm/day, 1–2 L/day; K^+ restriction to 60–70 mEq/day, phosphate restriction to keep plasma phosphorus < 4.5 mg/dL, magnesium restriction.
- Control of blood pressure with calcium channel blockers and betablockers.
- Treatment of anaemia with recombinant erythropoetin 50 units/kg once or twice a week.
- Maintenance of serum bicarbonate at 20 mEq/L by base supplement, i.e. sodium citrate, calcium carbonate, sodium bicarbonate.
- Reduction of water overload by diuretics; thiazides are ineffective when GFR is below 10 ml/min; hence loop diuretics are commonly used.
- Control of CHF with ACE inhibitors and angiotensin receptor blockers provided serum creatinine is < 3 mg%, else hyperkalemia and acidosis may worsen.
- Digoxin for CHF be used with caution since it is excreted by kidneys.
- Dihydroxy Vitamin D_3 0.25–0.5 µg daily along with calcium to lower plasma phosphorus and decrease parathyroid secretion and hence osteitis fibrosa cystica.
- Dialysis — haemodialysis usually three times a week or CAPD or CCPD.
- Kidney transplantation.

NEPHRITIC SYNDROME

- Edema, hypertension, haematuria, redcell casts, proteinuria (see Table 2.2).
- Mandatory laboratory investigations include complement levels, cryoglobulin, ASO titre, hepatitis panel, serum IgA, ANCA, anti GBM antibodies, C_3 nephritic factor.

- Encompasses (1) post infections glomerulonephritis, (2) IgA nephropathy and enock Schonlein Purpura, (3) ANCA associated GMN (small vessel vasculitides and Wegener's granulomatosis, (4) Anti GBM GMN and Goodpasture's syndrome (b) Cryoglobulin associated GMN.
- Renal biopsy should be considered. RPGN is likely when more than 50% glomeruli contain crescents. Electron microscopy shows subepithelial deposits in post streptococcal GMN due to trapped immune complexes, mesangial deposits of IgA in IgA nephropathy, granular deposits in subepithelium, subendothelium or mesangium in lupus nephritis, widening of basement membrane in Goodpasture's syndrome; but no deposits in Wegener's granulomatosis and PAN. Rapidly progressive GMN is likely when more than 50% glomeruli contain crescents. Nephritis of SLE, cryoglobulinemia, SABE, Goodpasture's syndrome and PAN usually belong to RPGN variety with rapid loss of renal function.
- *Treatment* includes aggressive reduction of hypertension and fluid overload and specific therapy for the underlying cause. Salt and water restriction, diuretic therapy and correction of electrolyte abnormalities are crucial. Penicillin for 10 days be used in post streptococcal GMN. IgA nephropathy can be treated with long term prednisolone orally with methyl prednisolone 1 gm/day IV for 3 days on months 1, 3, 5, and fish oil 2–5 gm daily. ANCA associated GMN is treated with prednisolone or methyl prednisolone and cyclophosphamide 1.5–2 mg/kg PO for 3 months. Plasma exchange and immunosuppressive therapy work well in Goodpasture's syndrome.

Table 2.2: **Differentiation of acute nephritic syndrome from nephrotic syndrome**

	Acute nephritic syndrome	Nephrotic syndrome
Previous illness	Preceding	No previous illness
Age	streptococcal infection	Most often seen in
	Predominantly school	pre-school child
	going child	
Onset	Sudden	Insidious
Oedema	Rarely severe	Presenting feature
		and rapidly becomes
		massive
Hypertension	Invariably present	Usually absent
Urine	Many red cells	Few red cells
Azotemia	Present	Absent
Recovery	In 90%	May occur
Death	Due to uremia or	Uremia may develop
	left ventricular	after months or years,
	failure.	Secondary infections
		common.

NEPHROTIC SYNDROME

Essentials of diagnosis

- Edema, hypoalbuminemia (serum albumin < 3 gm /dl)
- Gross albuminuria (protein excretion > 3.5 gm/1.73 m^2 per day).
- Dyspnoea due to pleural effusion, pulmonary edema, diaphragmatic compromise due to ascites.
- Loss of immunoglobulins in urine leading to increased propensity to infections, usually gram-positive organisms.
- Hyperlipidemia due to increased hepatic production of cholesterol and apo B and decreased clearance of VLDL.
- Decreased serum complement, vitamin D, zinc and copper.
- Loss of antithrombin III, protein C and S in urine leads to hypercoagulable state with renal vein thrombosis; highest incidence in membranous nephropathy.
- Fusion of foot process causes minimal change or lipoid nephrosis but when associated with C$_3$ and IgM deposits

it is due to focal and segmental glomerulosclerosis. In membranous nephropathy there is dense deposit in subepithelium; not responding to therapy in membrano proliferative form there is dense deposit in subendothelium.

* Renal biopsy is indicated in children not responding to therapy and in adults prior to therapy.

Treatment

* Prednisolone 1 mg/kg/day 4–6 weeks in children and upto 16 weeks in adults or till complete remission of proteinuria followed by gradual withdrawal. Patients with frequent relapse or steroid resistance need cyclophosphamide or chlorambucil. Best response is in minimal change disease.
* Supportive therapy — low salt diet, strict control of blood pressure, ACE inhibitors, high protein diet.

DISEASES WITH NEPHRITIC AND NEPHROTIC COMPONENTS

Renal involvement in SLE has 5 histologic patterns – type I (normal), type II (mesangial proliferative), type III (focal and segmental proliferative), type IV (diffuse proliferative), type V (membranous nephropathy). While type I and type II need no treatment, type III and type IV need aggressive immunosuppressive therapy. Type V when is superimposed on proliferative lesions needs treatment. Cyclophosphamide IV monthly for six months and then every 3 months for six doses is recommended along with methyl prednisolone 1gm IV daily for 3 doses and then oral prednisolone. Membranoproliferative (thick basement membrane) GMN has two forms – type I and type II. Type I is associated with upper respiratory infection with C_3, IgM, IgG deposit in granular pattern but in type II only there is C_3 deposit (C_3 nephritic factor). Type I presents with nephritic syndrome and less common type II with nephrotic syndrome. Treatment of both forms is with steroids along with antiplatelet drugs. Type II carries a less favorable prognosis and both forms recur after transplant, type II more commonly.

INTERSTITIAL NEPHRITIS

* Can be acute or chronic; acute disease usually associated with toxins or ischemia and mimics acute renal failure.
* In chronic form there is (1) reduced GFR, (2) hyperchloremic metabolic acidosis, (3) hyperkalemia, (4) decreased urinary concentrating ability, and (5) small contracted kidneys. Analgesics, urinary obstruction, vesicoureteric reflux, heavy metals, multiple myeloma and gout are usually responsible. Polyuria is characteristic and dehydration can occur due to salt wasting. Proteinuria is mild and urine may have broad waxy casts.
* Once there is evidence of interstitial fibrosis in biopsy, nothing can prevent progression to end stage renal disease.
* *Treatment* is that of primary cause, i.e. relief of obstruction, correction of VUR, discontinuation of analgesics etc.

POLYCYSTIC KIDNEY DISEASE (PKD)

* Autosomal dominant, age of onset 20–40 years.
* Flank pain with microscopic to gross haematuria, often mild proteinuria.
* History of urinary tract infection and urolithiasis.
* Hypertension, palpable renal mass (see Table 2.3).
* US shows more than 5 cysts distributed in cortex and medulla in each kidney.
* Often associated with pancreatic, hepatic, splenic cysts and cerebral aneurysms.

- No medical therapy can prevent development of renal failure but strict control of hypertension and low protein diet can delay the progression of the disease.

Table 2.3: Characteristic features of ADPKD and ARPKD

Features	ADPKD (adult type)	ARPKD (infantile type)
1. Inheritance pattern	Autosomal dominant	Autosomal recessive
2. Prevalence	1/400 to 1/1000	Rare
3. Age of onset	Usually adults	Neonates, children
4. Presentation	Loin pain, Hematuria, Infection of renal cysts	Abdominal mass, Renal failure, Failure to thrive
5. Hematuria	Common	May be present
6. Recurrent upper	Common urinary tract infection	May be present
7. Renal calculi	Common	Uncommon
8. Hypertension	Common	Common
9. Method of diagnosis	Ultrasound	Ultrasound
10. Renal size	Normal to very large	Large

MEDULLARY SPONGE KIDNEY

- Gross or microscopic haematuria, nephrolithiasis, recurrent urinary tract infection.
- Polyuria due to decreased urinary concentrating ability.
- IVU shows striations in papillary region due to accumulation of contrast in the dilated collecting ducts.
- *Treatment* is adequate fluid intake to prevent stone formation, thiazide diuretics to decrease calcium excretion if hypercalciuria is present, alkali therapy if there is renal tubular acidosis.

ACUTE PYELONEPHRITIS

- Fever, flank pain, shaking chills.
- Irritative voiding symptoms (urgency, frequency, dysuria).

- Pronounced costovertebral angle tenderness.
- UC may show hydronephrosis from stone or other source of obstruction.
- Urine culture is positive; varying degrees of haematuria with pyuria, bacteriuria; blood culture often positive.
- Empirical treatment prior to receipt of culture sensitivity is ampicillin 1 gm IV 6 hrly plus gentamicin 1 mg/kg IV 8 hrly, else ciprofloxacin 750 mg bid/ofloxacin 200 mg bid. IV antibiotics be continued for 1 day after patient becomes afebrile and oral preparation be then given. Duration of therapy is 14–21 days. Follow up urine culture is mandatory. Nephrostomy drainage may be required if there is ureteral obstruction.

ACUTE CYSTITIS

- Irritative voiding symptoms (dysuria, frequency, urgency).
- Suprapubic tenderness.
- Pyuria, bacteriuria, haematuria.
- Patient usually afebrile.
- Positive urine culture.
- *Treatment* is with ciprofloxacin 500 mg bid, norfloxacin 400 mg bid or ofloxacin 200 mg bid for 1–3 days.
- Symptomatic relief is with phenazopyridine 200 mg PO tid (Flavoxate).

PROSTATITIS

- Fever, irritative voiding symptoms.
- Perineal or suprapubic pain, often urinary obstruction and acute retention.
- Exquisitely tender prostate in PR examination; prostatic massage contraindicated for fear of causing septicemia.
- Positive urine culture.
- *Treatment* of acute bacterial prostatitis is as for acute pyelonephritis (see above).

- In chronic bacterial prostatitis (*E.coli*) fever is absent and symptoms are minimal. Patient may have low backpain; culture of prostatic massage specimen yields the organism. Treatment is with ciprofloxacin 500 mg/ofloxacin 200 mg bid for 1–3 months.
- Non bacterial prostatitis is the most common cause of prostatic syndrome and can be probably due to chlamydia, mycoplasma, ureaplasma and viruses and often autoimmune. Treatment is with NSAID along with empirical erythromycin 250 mg qid for 14 days.
- Prostatodynia, a noninflammatory disorder, has symptoms similar to chronic prostatitis. Patient may have hesitancy and interruption of flow. Often anal sphincter tone is increased and periprostatic tenderness may be present. It is likely due to pelvic floor musculature dysfunction or voiding dysfunction. Urodynamic testing may show voiding dysfunction (detrusor contraction without urethral relaxation, high urethral pressure). Treatment is with terazocin 1 mg/doxazocin 1 mg daily to releive bladder neck-urethral spasm. Pelvic floor dysfunction may respond to diazepam.

EPIDIDYMITIS

- Fever, irritative voiding symptoms.
- Pain at the tip of penis, urethral discharge, pain often referred to flanks.
- Scrotal swelling, tender epididymis; often prostatic tenderness.
- Urethral discharge may show gram -ve diplococci (gonococcus); white cells without organisms (chlamidya) – both transmitted sexually and varying degrees of pyuria, bacteriuria and haematuria in nonsexually transmitted variety.
- *Treatment* is with NSAID, scrotal elevation and antibiotics. In sexually transmitted form ceftriaxone

250 mg IM plus doxycycline 100 mg bid for 10 days is given; the sexual partner be also treated and the nonsexual form is treated as for chronic pyelonephritis.

INTERSTITIAL CYSTITIS

- Pain with bladder filling that is relieved by emptying.
- Often associated with urgency and frequency, nocturia.
- Negative urine culture.
- Submucosal petechiae in cystoscope; biopsy must be performed to exclude carcinoma, eosinophilic cystitis and tuberculous cystitis.
- *Treatment* is only symptomatic; amitriptyline, calcium channel blockers, pentosan polysulphate sodium, intravesical DMSO, BCG, hydrodistention can be tried.

BENIGN HYPERPLASIA OF PROSTATE (BPH)

Essentials of diagnosis

Obstructive or irritative voiding symptoms; obstructive symptoms include hesitancy, poor stream, double voiding, sensation of incomplete voiding, straining to urinate, post void dribbling; irritative symptoms include urgency, frequency and nocturia.

- Smooth firm enlarged prostate in PR, rectal mucosa free but size does not correlate with severity of symptoms or degree of obstruction.
- Can present as acute retention, haematuria, urinary tract infection, renal insufficiency.
- US can detect size, weight and nature of enlargement and can measure post-voiding volume.
- PSA estimation is necessary to exclude malignancy; urea creatinine and GFR estimation to exclude renal insufficiency.
- Cytometrogram, urodynamic studies and biopsy are optional.

Treatment

- Alphablockers – prazosin 1–5 mg bid, terazocin 1–10 mg daily, doxazosin – 1–8 mg daily, tamsulosin 0.4–0.8 mg daily.
- 5-alpha-reductase inhibitors — finasteride.
- Phytotherapy — plant extracts (speman).
- Minimally invasive surgery – transurethral needle ablation (TUNA), transurethral electrovaporization, high frequency focussed ultrasound, transurethral balloon dilatation, intraurethral stents, hyperthermia.
- Surgical procedures: Transurethral incision of prostate (TUIP), transurethral resection of prostate (TURP), prostatectomy.

RENAL CELL CARCINOMA

- Gross or microscopic haematuria.
- Flank pain or mass, cough and bone pain in metastatic disease.
- Systemic symptoms like fever, weight loss.
- Rarely erythrocytosis, hypercalcemia, Stauffer's syndrome (hepatic dysfunction in absence of metastasis)
- Solid renal mass in CT scan.
- *Treatment* is radical nephrectomy for localized tumors. T_3, T_4 or node positive patients can have adjuvant radiotherapy; metastatic disease can be given vinblastin, IL2 and alfa interferon but prognosis is poor.

TESTICULAR TUMOUR

- Painless enlargement of testis.
- Less common presentation is with acute testicular pain from intratesticular haemorrhage, secondary hydrocele, back pain from retroperitoneal metastasis, cough from pulmonary metastasis.
- Elevated hCG and alfa-fetoprotein in nonseminomas.

- Radical orchiectomy with irradiation is the treatment of choice for stage I and stage IIa (retroperitoneal disease < 10 cm) disease; for other advanced stages orchiectomy is combined with etoposide + cisplatin, often with bleomycin.

3

ENDOCRINE DISORDERS

HYPOPITUITARISM

- Sexual dysfunction, weakness, easy fatiguability; lack of resistance to stress, cold and fasting; axillary and pubic hair loss, infertility, diminished libido and erection.
- Low blood pressure, often visual defects due to pituitory tumours.
- Low free thyroxine, deficient cortisol response to cosyntropin, features of hypothyroidism.
- Low serum testosterone in men; amenorrhoea; low FSH, LH, elevated protactin.
- MRI may reveal a pituitary or hypothalamic lesion – Hypopituitarism without a mass lesion may be idiopathic or may be caused by trauma, encephalitis, autoimmunity, hemochromatosis, stroke etc. Clinical manifestations depend upon which specific hormone in lacking and whether the deficiency is partial or complete.
- Transsphenoidal removal of pituitary lesion may reverse the symptoms but postoperative hyponatremia may occur. Prolactin excess can be managed by dopamine agonists. Octreotide may be effective for GH secretory tumours. Radiation therapy with x-ray, gamma knife, heavy particles may be necessary. Life time hormone replacement therapy with corticosteroids, thyroxine, sex hormones (androgen, estrogen, hCG (for spermatogenesis) and growth hormone.

DIABETES INSIPIDUS

- Polyuria (2–20 L/day), polydipsia, craving for ice water.
- Urine specific gravity < 1006.

- Vasopressin reduces urine output; can present as hypernatremia and dehydration, especially after hypothalamic damage due to shock/anoxia.
- Hyperuricemia indicates central diabetes insipidus.
- MRI be done to find out pathology in brain-in and around pituitary; absence of T1 bright spot in posterior pituitary is suggestive of central diabetes insipidus.
- *Treatment* is by desmopressin, 100 µg/ml sol, intranasally 12–24 hours as per need or SC/IM/IV 1–4 µg every 12 hours; oral dose is 0.1 mg daily increased to maximum of 0.2 mg every 8 hours.
  Hydrochlorthiazide 50–100 mg/day with potassium supplement or amiloride; indomethacin 50 mg tid, indomethacin-desmopressin combination are effective in central and nephrogenic diabetes insipidus.

ACROMEGALY

Essentials of diagnosis

- Prognathism (jaw protrusion), large feet and hands.
- Coarsening of facial features, deep voice, macroglossia.
- Soft doughy sweaty headshake; carpal tunnel syndrome.
- Amenorrhoea, headache, field defects, weakness, sweating.
- Increased IGF-I; serum GH not suppressed by glucose
- Hypertension, hyperglycemia; decreased libido, irregular menses, impotency.
- Tufting of terminal phalanges; CT-MRI demonstrates pituitary tumor.

Treatment

- Transsphenoidal removal of tumor.
- Dopamine agonist cabergoline 1–1.75 mg/week orally, quinagolide — 0.075 mg/d PO increased upto 0.6 mg PO/d.

- Octreotide 20 mg – 40 mg IM per month to maintain serum GH of 1 ng – 2.5 n/ml.
- GH receptor antagonist – pegvisomant 20 mg daily for 12 weeks.
- Stereotactic radiosurgery who fail after microsurgery and medications.

HYPERPROLACTINEMIA

- Men — hypogonadism, decreased libido, erectile dysfunction, infertility.
- Women — amenorrhoea-oligomenorrhoea, galactorrhoea, infertility.
- Raised serum prolactin (≥250 ng/ml).
- MRI demonstrates the adenoma.
- Large tumors may cause headache, visual symptoms, and pituitary insufficiency.
- *Treatment* (a) dopamine agonist – cabergoline 0.25 mg PO once a week raised to 0.5 mg twice a week. Alternatively bromocriptine 1.25 – 20 mg/d orally or pergolide 0.125 – 2 mg/d orally, or quinagolide (see above); (b) trans-sphenoidal surgery for large tumors compromising visual fields or non responders·to dopamine agonists; (c) Gammaknife/conventional radiotherapy.

THYROID NODULES

- Single or multiple thyroid nodules can be only found after careful palpation from behind in a sitting patient. As the patient swallows water, thyroid nodules may be perceived moving beneath the fingers.
- Neck should be examined for lymphadenopathy, auscultation should be made for bruit, hypo/hyper thyroid state be confirmed.
- Thyroid function tests (T_3, T_4, TSH, antithyroid antibiodies) be done routinely.

- Ultrasound examination may help to know nodule to be cystic (benign) or solid (malignant) and helps in biopsy.
- FNAC of nodule is mandatory.
- High index of suspicion be for nodules appearing after head and neck radiation, associated vocal cord palsy, lymphadenopathy in neck, nodules with punctate calcification, cold nodules in ^{123}I scan.
- Non palpable thyroid nodules can be detected in US, CT, MRI but only when more than 1.5 cm be biopsied. Microscopic "micropapillary" carcinoma if discovered is a variant of normal.

MULTINODULAR GOITER

- Common in areas of iodine deficiency; high rate of congenital hypothyroidism and cretinism.
- Most are euthyroid and some are hypothyroid.
- If substernal can cause respiratory distress, dysphagia, SVC obstruction, Horner's syndrome, bleeding form esophageal varices, phrenic/recurrent laryngeal palsy, and often pleural/pericardial effusion.
- Addition of potassium iodide to table salt greatly reduces the prevalence of endemic goiter and cretinism.

HYPOTHYROIDISM

- Weakness, fatigue, cold intolerance, constipation, weight gain, depression, menorrhagia, hoarseness.
- Thinning of hair, pallor, brittle nails, diminished auditory acuity, dry skin.
- Thick tongue, thinning of outer half of eyebrows, pleuropericardial effusion, bradycardia, cardiomegaly, hypothermia.
- Delayed tendon reflexes, hyponatremia, hypoglycemia, ↑ cholesterol.
- Low T_4 and low radio-iodine uptake.

- TSH elevated in primary hypothyroidism (see Table 3.1).
- Titers of antibodies against thyroperoxidase and thyroglobulin are high in patient of Hashimotos' thyroiditis.
- *Treatment* is with levothyroxine 50–100 µg daily; older people or those with CAD be given 25 µg daily, then raised gradually.
- Treatment of myxedema coma is with levothyroxine 400 µg IV followed by 100 µg IV daily, prevention of hypothermia, hypoglycemia, hyponatremia, treatment of precipitating infection, and hydrocortisone 100 mg IV followed by 25–50 mg tid.

Table 3.1: Difference between primary and secondary hypothyroidism

Features	*Primary* hypothyroidism	*Secondary* hypothyroidism
1. Skin	Coarse	Soft and silky
2. Blood pressure	Hypertension or normal	Hypotension or normal
3. Menstrual cycle	Menorrhagia	Amenorrhoea
4. Trans-cardiac diameter	Increased	Normal, decreased
5. Serum choleserol	Increased	Decreased
6. Serum choleserol	Increased	Not altered
7. Evidence of deficiency of other pituitiary hormones	Absent	Present

HYPERTHYROIDISM

- Sweating, weight loss, anxiety, diarrhoea, heat intolerance, irritability, weakness, menstrual irregularity.
- Tachycardia, warm moist skin, tremor, stare and lid lag, angina, often osteoporosis.
- In Grave's disease: goiter often with bruit; ophthalmopathy (chemosis, proptosis, diplopia). (Table 3.2).

- ↑ T3, ↑ T4, ↑ TSH receptor antibodies; ↑ radioiodine uptake. MRI documents Grave's ophthalmopathy.
- *Treatment* is with (1) propranolol 20–80 mg QID, (2) neomercazole 30–60 mg daily, propylthiouracil 300–600 mg daily, (3) iodinated agents, (4) radioactive iodine (for those above reproductive age or not wanting further children), (5) surgery (particularly when there is suspicion of malignancy), (6) prednisolone 40–60 mg/d for ophthalmopathy or low dose 20 Gy to each orbit over 2 weeks.

Table 3.2: Differential diagnosis of Grave's disease and toxic nodular goiter

	Grave's disease	*Toxic nodular goiter*
Age	Younger	Older
Gland	Smooth, diffuse enlargement	Nodular, irregular
Eye signs	Common	Rare
Cardiac involvement	Uncommon	Common
Pressure symptoms	Uncommon	Common
Autoimmune disease	Common	Uncommon

THYROIDITIS

- Thyromegaly-painful in acute and subacute forms and painless in chronic form.
- Associated Sjogren's syndrome and myasthenia gravis in Hashimoto's lymphotrophic thyroiditis; often polyglandular autoimmunity with multiple hormone deficiency.
- Initial hyperthyroidism due to release of stored T_3, T_4 but ultimately hypothyroidism develops.
- Antithyroid peroxide and antithyroglobulin antibodies in Hashimoto's thyroditis.
- De Quervain's thyroiditis (granulomatous and giant cell thyroiditis) is of acute onset but with low iodine uptake, high ESR and normal antithyroid antibodies.
- Riedel's thyroiditis (woody or invasive fibrous thyroiditis) may cause hypothyroidism as well as

hypoparathyroidism. Gland is stony hard and adherent to deeper structures causing dysphagia, dyspnoea, hoarseness often associated with retroperitoneal fibrosis, fibrosing mediastinitis and biliary sclerosis.

* *Treatment* of Hashimoto's thyroiditis is with aspirin and levothyroxine (if hypothyroid) and that of Riedel's thyroiditis with long term tamoxifen supplemented with hydrocortisone.

HYPOPARATHYROIDISM

* Tetany, carpopedal spasms, tingling of lips and hands, muscle and abdominal cramps, psychologic changes, Parkinsonism.
* Positive Chvostek's sign, and Trousseau's phenomenon, defective nails and teeth, cataracts, hyperactive tendon reflexes.
* Low serum calcium, high serum phosphate, normal alkaline phosphatase; reduced calcium excretion; low serum magnessium.
* CT – basal ganglia calcification, dense bones.
* *Treatment* is with oral calcium 1–3 gm daily with 1,25 dihydroxy vit D_3 0.25 µg daily or Vit D_2 (ergocalciferol) 25,000 units daily or 25 hydroxy vitamin D_3 (calcifediol) 20 µg daily or dihydrotachysterol 0.125 mg–1 mg daily along with magnesium oxide 600 mg daily. Transplantation of cryopreserved parathyroid tissue may be attempted.

HYPERPARATHYROIDISM

* Renal stones, often recurrent; polyuria, constipation, hypertension, fatigue, mental changes.
* Bone pain, often cystic changes and pathologic fracture.
* Raised serum and urine calcium; high urine phosphate, low to normal serum phosphate, normal to increased alkaline phosphatase.

- Increased level of parathyroid hormone, loss of cortical bone and gain of trabecular bone.
- Symptoms are with "bones, stones, abdominal groans, psychic moans, with fatigue over tones".
- Tc peretechnate subtraction scintigraphy/Tc 99 sestamibi, US, MRI can detect the enlarged parathyroids/ectopic parathyroid tissue.
- *Treatment* (a) hypercalcemia is treated with increased fluid intake, bisphosphonates- zolendronate 2–4 mg or palmidronate 30–90 mg IV. (b) Parathyroidectomy for parathyroid bone disease/stone disease, cortical bone density ≥25D below normal, high calcium excretion.

OSTEOPOROSIS

- Asymptomatic to severe backache from vertebral fracture
- Loss of height, spontaneous fractures
- Demineralisation, especially of spine, hip and pelvis
- Normal levels of serum parathyroid hormone, vit D, calcium, phosphorus and alkaline phosphatase
- CT densitometry for vertebral demineralization and dual energy X-ray absorptiometry (DEXA) for any bone.
- *Treatment* is with (1) estrogen replacement for postmenopausal women; (2) bisphosphonates – alendronate 10 mg orally daily or IV pamidronate/zolendronate every 3 month; (3) selective estrogen receptor modulator (SERM), e.g. raloxifene 60 mg PO daily (unlike estrogen it does hot reduce hot flushes but relieves vaginal dryness, and increases bone density without causing endometrial hyperplasia, uterine bleeding or cancer or breast soreness); (4) calcitonin 200 IU nasal puff daily; (5) calcium and Vit D supplement.

OSTEOMALACIA

- Painful proximal muscle weakness (especially pelvic girdle), bone pain and tenderness

- Decreased bone density from diminished mineralization of osteoid.
- Increased alkaline phosphatase, decreased Vitamin D_3, hypocalcemia, hypocalciuria, hypophosphatemia, secondary hyperparathyroidism.
- *Treatment* is with adequate sunlight exposure, Vitamin D supplement along with calcium, discontinuation of aluminum containing antacids, oral phosphate supplement, growth hormone supplement.

PAGET'S DISEASE

- Bone pain, kyphosis, bowed tibias, large head, headache, deafness, increased warmth over involved bone
- Normal serum calcium and phosphorus, markedly raised alkaline phosphatase, increased hydroxyproline excretion.
- X-ray-involved bone denser and thicker, osteoporosis circumscripta in skull bones; Technetium pyrophosphate bone scan may show increased bone activity; fissure fractures.
- *Treatment* is with (a) bisphosphonates – tiludronate 400 mg PO daily, alendronate 20–40 mg orally daily or 70 mg once weekly, risedronate 30 mg PO daily, etidronate 300 mg PO daily; (b) nasal calcitonin spray 200 IU daily.

ADDISON'S DISEASE

- Weakness, low blood pressure, sparse axillary hair, anorexia, weight loss, easy fatiguability, small heart.
- Increased skin pigmentation especially of creases, pressure areas, nipples, elbows, knees and knuckles.
- Low serum sodium, raised potassium, calcium and urea, neutropenia, mild anaemia, eosinophilia, relative lymphocytosis
- Raised plasma ACTH, low plasma cortisol that fails to rise after corticotropin.

- CT scan – small noncalcified adrenals in autoimmune Addison's disease; calcification in adrenals in tuberculosis, adrenal haemorrhage; enlarged adrenals in granulomatous disease.
- *Treatment* is with replacement therapy (a) hydrocortisone 15–25 mg daily; (b) fludrocortisone 0.05–0.3 mg daily (if postural hypotension); (c) DHEA 50 mg daily to women. In adrenoleukodystrophy – "Lorenzo oil" normalizes serum very long chain fatty acids but not symptoms which may improve following haematopoietic stem cell transplantation.

CUSHING'S SYNDROME

- Central obesity, muscle wasting, thin skin, easy bruisability, psychologic changes, hirsutism, purple striae, moon face, buffalo hump.
- Osteoporosis, hypertension, poor wound healing.
- Hyperglycemia, glycosuria, leukocytosis, lymphocytopenia, hypokalemia.
- Avascular bone necrosis, acne, glaucoma.
- Elevated serum cortisol and urinary free cortisol, lack of normal supression by dexamethasone.
- *Treatment* (a) transsphenoidal resection of pituitary adenoma with hydrocortisone supplement for 3–6 months or till normal corticotrophs regain function; (b) if no relief laparoscopic bilateral adrenalectomy or gamma knife; (c) ketoconazole 200 mg qid for those who are not surgical candidates and in metastatic adrenal carcinoma/unresectable adrenal carcinoma; (d) mitotane and metyrapone are used in hypercorticolism of unresectable adrenal carcinoma.

HIRSUTISM AND VIRILIZATION

- Menstrual disorders, acne, increased muscularity, androgenic alopecia, deepening of voice, enlargement

of clitoris, anovulation, defeminization (decrease in breast size, loss of feminine adipose tissue).
- Occasionally a palpable pelvic tumor.
- Urinary 17 ketosteroid and serum DHEAS and androstenodione increased in adrenal disorders.
- Serum testosterone often elevated.
- *Treatment* (a) drugs causing hirsutism be stopped; (b) postmenopausal women with severe hyperandrogenism should have bilateral oophorectomy (provided CT scan of adrenal and ovaries are normal) since small hilar tumor of ovary are often invisible; (c) spironolactone 50–100 mg twice daily on days 5–25 of menstrual cycle; (d) cyproterone acetate 2 mg daily along with oral contraceptive; (e) finasteride 5 mg daily or flutamide 250 mg daily; (f) metformin 500–1000 mg twice daily in polycystic ovarian disease; (g) local treatment — depilatories, electrolysis. Antiandrogen drugs be given only to nonpregnant women and they be given OCP to prevent pregnancy since use during pregnancy causes malformations and pseudo-hermaphroditism in male infants.

HYPERALDOSTERONISM

- Hypertension, polyuria, polydipsia, muscular weakness often mimicking periodic paralysis.
- Alkalosis, hypokalemia.
- Elevated plasma (>20 μg/dL) and urine aldosterone levels (> 20 μg/day) and low plasma renin level (< 5 μg/dl).
- *Treatment* (a) bilateral adrenal hyperplasia is treated with spironolactone; bilateral adrenalectomy corrects the hypokalemia but not hypertension; (b) laparoscopic adrenalectomy for unilateral adrenal adenoma.

PHEOCHROMOCYTOMA

- Attacks of headache, palpitations, perspiration.

- Hypertension, frequently sustained but often paroxysmal.
- Attacks of nausea, abdominal pain, chest pain, weakness, dyspnoea, tremor, visual disturbances.
- Anxiety, tremor, weight loss, heat intolerance.
- Elevated urinary catecholamines or their metabolites. Urinary metanephrine above 2.2 mg per mg of creatinine and more than 135 mg total catecholamine per gram of creatinine.
- Normal T_3, T_4.
- *Treatment* is laparoscopic removal of tumor after preoperative blood pressure control by phenoxybenzamine 10 mg bid and propranolol 10–40 mg 4 times daily.

MALE HYPOGONADISM

- Diminished libido and erection.
- Decreased growth of body hair, testes may be small or normal.
- Decreased serum testosterone.
- Increased FSH and LH in testicular failure (hypergonadotropic hypogonadism); decreased FSH and LH in hypogonadotropic hypogonadism (pituitary failure)
- Klinefelter's syndrome (seminifero tubule dysgenesis) or 47 XXY is most common form, small fibrotic firm testes with tall stature, gynaecomastia, azoospermia.
- A failure in testicular secretion of testosterone causes rise in LH. When testicular Sertoli cell function is deficient FSH is elevated. Testicular failure occurs in mumps, irradiation, cancer chemotherapy, autoimmunity, myotonic dystrophy, Kline felter's syndrome, etc.
- Men with gynaecomastia may be screened for partial 17 ketosteroid reductase deficiency in which androstenedione and estrone are elevated. If prolactin

is normal, MRI of pituitary be done to exclude tumor or granuloma.

- Before treating hypogonadism in men over 40, prostate cancer be excluded. Testosterone (enanthate or cypionate) 200 mg IM every 2 weeks or 300 mg every 3 weeks or oral fluoxymesterone or methyl testosterone, or testosterone skin patch 5 mg/d or gel 5 gm (500 mg testosterone) daily are sufficient.

DIABETES MELLITUS

Essentials of diagnosis

1. Type I diabetes

- Polyuria, polydipsia, and rapid weight loss associated with random plasma glucose $\geq$ 200 mg/dl.
- Ketonemia, ketonuria or both.
- Fasting plasma glucose $\geq$ 126 mg/dl after overnight fast in 2 or more occasion.

2. Type II diabetes

- Most patients are above 40 years and obese
- Polyuria, polydipsia, ketonuria and weight loss generally uncommon; often asymptomatic (see Table 3.3).
- Candidal vaginitis in women; hypertension, dyslipidemia, cataract, paresthesia, atherosclerosis are often associated.
- Fasting plasma glucose $\geq$ 126 mg/dl after overnight fast on 2 or more occasions or more than 200 mg/dl 2 hours after 75 gm glucose.

3. Maturity onset diabetes of the young

Autosomal dominant, occurring in nonobese young due to impaired glucose – induced secretion of insulin.

4. Diabetes mellitus associated with mutation of mitochondrial DNA

Maternally transmitted mild type II diabetes often with hearing loss, and MELAS (myopathy, encephalopathy, lactic acidosis and stroke like episodes).

5. Obesity with diabetes

Waist to hip ratio above 0.9 in men and above 0.8 in women are associated with increased risk of diabetes. Diabetes should be suspected in women with chronic candidal vulvovaginitis, as well as those with recurrent fetal loss, polyhydramnios, large babies, preeclampsia, etc.

Table 3.3: General characteristics of IDDM and NIDDM

Features	IDD	NIDDM
1. Genetic locus	Chromosome 6	Unknown; in MODY, Chromosome 7
2. Age of onset	<40 yrs	>40 yrs
3. Body weight	Normal to wasted	Obese
4. Plasma insulin	Low or absent	Normal or high
5. Plasma glucose	High, suppressible	High, resistant
6. Acute complication	Ketoacidosis	Hyperosmolar
7. Insulin therapy	Responsive	Responsive or resistant
8. Sulfonylurea therapy	Unresponsive	Responsive
9. Auto antibodies	Present	Absent
10. Early death without treatment	Yes	No
11. Other autoimmune disease	Present	Absent

Laboratory diagnosis

- Glucosuria as detected in the paper strip impregnated with glucose oxidase and a chromogen system. A normal renal threshold for glucose as well as reliable bladder emptying is essential for interpretation.

- Ketonuria detected by nitroprusside test but it does not detect β-hydroxybutyric acid.
- ↑ Fasting, postprandial blood sugar and positive GTT after 75 gm oral glucose.
- ↑ Glycosylated haemoglobin; Normal Hb A_{IC} is 4–6%; HbA_{Ia} + HbA_{Ib} is 2–4% of total haemoglobin. Their levels reflect glycemic control over past 8–12 weeks.
- ↑ Serum fructosamine level; indicates ghycemic control over past 2 weeks.

Treatment

- Diet – balanced nutritious diet; if obese, caloric restriction to 1600–1800 kCal/d. Limit carbohydrate intake by substituting noncholestrerologenic monounsaturated oils like olive oil or rapeseed oil. Daily total cholesterol intake be < 300 mg; protein 10–12% of total calories with saturated fat < 8–9%, PUFA 8–9%, fiber 20–35 gm; rest calories being from monounsaturated fat and carbohydrates. Artificial sweetners (aspartame) may be used in place of sucrose; sorbitol and fructose are nutritive sweetners.
- Oral hypoglycemic agents (OHA).
  Tolbutamide 0.5–2 gm in 2–3 divided doses, tolazamide 0.1–1 gm in two divided doses, glyburide 1.25–20 mg in two doses, glipizide 2.5–40 mg in 1–2 doses, glimeperide 1–4 mg single dose, gliclazide 40–120 mg in two divided doses, glibenclamide 5–20 mg in two divided doses are the sulphonyl urea derivatives that have insulinotropic effect on pancreas. They bind to a receptor that closes ATP sensitive potassium channel on pancreatic betacell there by depolarizing the cell membrane leading to influx of extracellular calcium that facilitates exocytosis of insulin granules.
- Non sulphonyl urea OHA are repaglinide given as 4 mg in two divided doses and nateglinide 60–120 mg tid. Both are short acting and when given before meals prevent post prandial glucose rise.

- Biguanides that improves glucose utilization is metformin, dose is 5–1 gm bid.
- Thiazolidinediones are insulin sesitizers given as – rosiglitazone 4–8 mg daily, and pioglitazone 15–45 mg daily as single dose.
- Alfaglucosidase inhibitors are acarbose and miglitol both given as 75–300 mg in 3 divided doses with first bite of food.

Insulin

Insulin is indicated for type I diabetes as well as for type II diabetes who poorly respond to diet and OHA. It can be (1) ultrashort acting – insulin lispro and insulin aspart; (2) short acting – regular insulin (human/pork); (3) intermediate acting – lente, NPH; (4) long acting – ultralente, insulin glargine. Premixed insulins – regular with NPH as 30:70 and 50:50 are also available. In insulin lispro aminoacids lysine and proline are interchanged in B_{28} and B_{29} positions; while in insulin aspart proline replaces aspartic acid at B_{28}. When injected SC they quickly dissociate to monomers and are rapidly absorbed. Effect starts 20 minutes after injection, unlike 60 minutes taken by regular insulin. Lente insulin is a mixture of 30% semilente with 70% ultralente, both complexed to zinc ions. NPH is two parts soluble crystalline zinc insulin with 1 part protamine zinc insulin. Insulin glargine is a clear insulin in which asparagine at position 21 is replaced by glycine and two arginines are added to betachain thus raising the isoelectric point to neutral. Neutral protamine lispro (NPH) premixed with insulin lispro is also available and can be given within 15 minutes of starting the meal.

1 unit of regular insulin is needed for every 15 gram excess intake of carbohydrate. Dawn phenomenon is morning hyperglycemia due to cortisol surge but in Somogyi effect morning hyperglycemia is due to hypoglycemia during sleep. In the former insulin evening dose is to be increased and in the latter the dose is to be decreased.

Essentials of diagnosis

- Hyperadrenergic symptoms – tremor, tremulousness, tachycardia, sweating, extreme weakness, full bounding pulse.
- Neurologic dysfunction-confusion, delirium, coma, convulsion, blurred vision, diplopia, headache, slurred speech.
- Fasting hypoglycemia in an otherwise healthy well nourished adult is mostly due to insulinoma.
- Diagnosis of hypoglycemia of insulinoma is by Whipple's triad of (a) hypoglycemic symptoms, (b) blood glucose below 50 mg%, (c) prompt recovery with glucose.
- In insulinoma proinsulin level may be 30–90% of total serum immunoreactive insulin (most specific).
- Glucagon IV 1 mg causes inappropriate insulin rise in insulinoma (> 200 IU/ml)
- Localisation of insulinoma is by contrast MRI, hepatic vein insulin sampling while delivering calcium to suspected pancreatic segment by selective arteriography.

Treatment

- 20% dextrose, 50 ml, rapid IV followed by 10% dextrose IV drip.
- Glucagon 1 mg IV.
- If insulinoma suspected surgery be performed.

Hyperglycemic hyperosmolar state (nonketotic hyperglycemic coma)

Essentials of diagnosis

- Hyperglycemia > 600 mg/dl
- Serum osmolality > 310 mosm/kg
- No acidosis; pH > 7.3
- Serum bicarbonate > 15 m Eq/L
- Normal anion gap (< 14 m Eq/L)
- Severe dehydration, polyuria, polydipsia

Treatment

- Rapid IV saline upto 4–6 litres in 8–10 hrs to combat hypovolemia and oliguria; else 0.45% saline. Once blood sugar reaches 250 mg/dl fluid replacement be by 0.45% saline, 5% dw to maintain blood sugar between 250–300 mg/dl to reduce risk of cerebral edema.
- Insulin therapy – 15 units IV, then 15 units SC every 4 hours.
- Potassium and phosphate replacement.

Diabetic ketoacidosis

- Hyperglycemia > 250 mg/dl; glycosuria
- Acidosis; pH < 7.3, - anion gap

Table 3.4: Difference in coma due to hypoglycaemia and ketoacidosis

	Hypoglycaemic coma	Coma with ketosis
History	No food intake; exercise	Too little or no insulin, or unaccustomed infection or digestive disturbances
Onset	In good previous health; related to last insulin injection	Ill health for several days
Symptoms	Hypoglycaemia; occasional vomiting from depot insulins	Of glycosuria and dehydration; abdominal pain and vomiting
Signs	Moist skin and tongue Full pulse Normal or raised BP Intraocular pressure-normal Shallow or normal breathing Brisk reflexes	Dry skin and tongue Weak pulse Low blood pressure Decreased Air hunger Diminished reflexes
Urine	No ketonuria No glycosuria, if bladder recently emptied	Ketonuria Glycosuria
Blood	Hypoglycaemia (<60mg/dl). Normal plasma bicarbonate	Hyperglycaemia (>300 mg/dl). Reduced plasma bicarbonate

- Serum bicarbonate - < 15 mEq/L
- Raised ketones in serum.
- Polyuria, polydipsia, vomiting, fruity breath odor, rapid deep breathing, hypotension, tachycardia, abdominal pain, hypothermia, leukocytosis in absence of infection.

Treatment

- Rapid fluid replacement with 0.9% saline; 4–5 litres may be required.
- IV sodibicarb till pH reaches 7.1.
- IV potassium and phosphate replacement form 3rd bottle of saline onwards, avoid hyperkalemia.
- IV insulin 0.1 unit/kg loading, then 0.1 unit/kg/hr by infusion till blood sugar falls to 250 mg/dl when SC insulin may be given along with 5% dextrose.
- Control of infection, prevention of renal failure.

Lactic acidosis

- Severe acidosis with hyperventilation
- Blood pH < 7.3, bicarbonate < 15 mEq/L.
- Anion gap > 15; absent ketones
- Serum lactate > 5 mmol/L.
- *Treatment* is (1) IV bicarbonate to keep pH above 7.2; (2) aggressive treatment of sepsis/hypoperfusion state; (3) maintenance of adequate oxygenation and vascular perfusion; (4) haemodialysis, if large sodium load of IV bicarbonate is unacceptable.

Hyperlipedemia

- Associated with obesity, diabetes, hypothyroidism, nephrotic syndrome.
- Diuretics and OCP increase total cholesterol and triglycerides; beta blockers increase total cholesterol and decrease HDL.

- Hyperlipidemia enhances atherosclerosis of coronary, cerebral, renal and limb vessels; produces xanthoma, xanthelsma, pancreatitis and hepatosplenomegaly.
- Total cholesterol is HDL + VLDL + LDL cholesterol.
- LDL cholesterol is = Total cholesterol – HDL – triglyceride/5 (VLDL)
- There is no normal range for serum lipids as it varies from population to population.
- Levels of cholesterol lowering is definitely beneficial in CAD.
- TG reduction is best achieved with niacin, gemfibrozil, simvastatin and atorvastatin; LDL reduction with atorvastatin, fluvastatin, simvastatin, lovastatin, pravastatin; and HDL rise with niacin, and gemfibrozil.
- Doses of lipid modifying drugs is atorvastatin 10–80 mg OD; fluvastatin 20–40 mg OD, gemfibrozil 600–1200 mg OD/two divided doses, pravastatin 20–40 mg OD, simvastatin 10–80 mg OD, niacin 100 mg OD to 3 gm in divided doses; cholestipol 5–30 gm in two divided doses, gugulip bd, fenofibrate, benzafibrate and omega-3 fatty acids.

4

DISEASES OF LUNGS AND RESPIRATION

BRONCHIAL ASTHMA

Essentials of diagnosis

- Episodic or chronic wheezing, breathlessness, dry cough and chest tightness.
- Symptoms frequently worse at night or early morning
- Diffuse chronic and prolonged expiration on examination of chest.
- Obstructive pattern in PFT with partial or complete reversibility with bronchodilators.
- Positive bronchial provocation challenge.
- Exclude bronchopulmonary aspergillosis, vasculitides, tropical eosinophilia, GE reflux, cardiac asthma, laryngomalacia (Table 4.1).

Table 4.1: Differentiation of cardiac asthma from bronchial asthma

	Cardiac asthma	Bronchial asthma
1. Past history	Of hypertension, aortic disease or IHD	Of previous attacks of asthma or other allergic conditions
2. Age	Onset usually after 40	Any age
3. Precipitating factor	May be precipitated by exertion or acute myocardial infarction or hypertension	Trigger factors may be infection, be infection, non-specific irritants, external allergens, exercise or emotional factors

	Cardiac asthma	Bronchial asthma
4. Symptoms		
a. Cough	Cough and dyspnoea almost simultaneous. Pink frothy sputum which increases in intensity towards end of attack	Starts with dyspnoea Expectoration of thick sticky sputum
b. Wheezing	Rare	Usual
c. Sweating	Prominent	Rare unless acute severe asthma
Signs		
a. Inspection:		
i. Accessory ms. of respiration	Not active	Active
ii. Shape of chest	Normal	Emphysematous
iii. Respirations	Rapid and shallow	Rapid with prolonged expiration
b. Auscultation:		
i. Chest	Expiration not unduly prolonged Rales more than rhonchi In early stages at long bases, gradually ascending up with progress of the attack	Expiration markdly prolonged Rhonchi more than rales Signs diffuse all over the lungs
ii. Heart	A_2 may be loud Left ventricular gallop	Normal A_2 RV gallop late feature of severe bronchial asthma
c. Pulse	Full and bounding,or pulsus alternans	Feeble and rapid
d. B.P.	Usually elevated	Normal or low
e. Extremities	Cold	Warm (with CO_2 retention)
f. Signs of underlying disease	AR, AS, hypertension, or IHD	No evidence of cardiovascular disease

	Cardiac asthma	*Bronchial asthma*

6. Investigation:
   ECG
   CXR.
	LV preponderance,
	acute MI or LBBB
	Hilae become hazy,
	'bat's wing' shadowing
	if pulmonary oedema
		Normal or RV
		preponderance
		Normal or
		hyperinflated lungs
		Focal or segmental
		atelactasis due to
		mucus plugs

Asthma can be extrinsic or intrinsic (Table 4.2)

Table 4.2: Features of extrinsic and intrinsic asthma

Extrinsic asthma	*Intrinsic asthma*

Clinical features:
1. Young patient- child
   or teenager
2. History of eczema in
   childhood
3. Family history of
   asthma, eczema or hay fever
4. Attacks related to
   specific antigens.
5. Intermittent attacks
6. Attacks are acute but
   usually self limiting
7. Not aspirin-sensitive,
   occasional polyps
	1. Adult patient over 35 or more
	
	2. No history of eczema
	   in childhood
	3. Negative family history
	
	4. Attacks related to infection,
	   exercise, etc.
	5. Often persistent asthma
	6. Attacks more fulminant and
	   severe
	7. Aspirin-sensitive, nasal
	   polyps

Investigations: 1. Skin test usually+ve 2. IgE frequently raised	1. Skin test usually-ve. 2. Normal or low IgE.
Response to treatment: Good response to beta-agonists and sodium cromoglycate. Prognosis favourable.	Poor response to beta-agonists variable response to cromoglycate Prognosis poor.

Treatment

Treatment depends upon severity of asthma i.e.

Mild – PEF/FEV_1 > 80% predicted

Moderate – PEF/FEV$_1$ – 60–80% with variability of $\geq$ 30%.
Severe – PEF/FEV$_1$ - < 60% predicted with variability
$\leq$ 30%.

Mild asthma

a. For quick relief – Inhaled β_2 agonist.
b. Long term control – Inhaled low dose corticosteroid or cromolyn or nedocromil or sustained release theophylline.

Moderate asthma

a. Quick relief – Inhaled β_2 agonist or nebulisation.
b. Long term control – Inhaled medium dose corticosteroid with sustained release theophylline or long acting oral β_2 agonist.

Severe asthma

a. Quick relief – Inhaled/nebulised β_2 agonists or IV β_2 agonists.
b. Long term control – Inhaled high dose corticosteroid and long acting β_2 agonists with oral corticosteroid 2 mg/kg/day or methyl prednisolone 0.5–1 mg/kg IV every 6 hours, changed to oral steroid subsequently.

Quick relief medications for asthma

1. Salbutamol/ albuterol	90–100 µg/puff – 2 puffs every 4–6 hours or 1.25–5 mg in normal saline nebulised every 4–8 hours
2. Bioterol	370 µg/puff, 2–3 puffs every 6–8 hours or 0.25–5 mg nebulization every 4–8 hour
3. Pirbuterol	200 µg/puff, 2 puffs every 4–6 hours

4. Salmeterol   250 µg/puff 2 puffs twice daily
5. Formoterol
6. Orciprenaline   400 µg/puff 2–4 puffs 4–6 hourly
7. Terbutaline   250 µg/puff, 2–4 puffs 4–6 hourly

Long term medications for asthma

1. *Steroids*

Beclomethasone	40 µg/puff, 2–3 puffs twice daily
Budesonide	100 µg/puff, two puffs twice daily
Flunisolide	250 µg/puff, 2–4 puffs twice daily
Fluticasone	110–220 µg/puff, 2 puffs of 110 µg twice daily
Triamcinolone	100 µg/puff, 2–3 puffs 4 times daily

2. *Mastcell stabilizers*

Cromolyn	800 µg/puff, 2–4 puffs 4 times daily or 20 mg nebulised 4 times daily
Sodium chromglycate	1 mg/puff – 2 puffs 4–6 times daily
Nedocromil	1.75 mg/puff, 2 puffs 4 times daily
Ketotifen	1 mg tab, 1–2 tables PO twice daily

3. *Anticholinergics*

Ipratropium	18 µg/puff, 2–4 puffs 6 hourly or 0.25–0.5 mg nebulised every 6 hours

4. *Leukotrine modifiers*

Monteleukast	10 mg PO once daily
Zafirlukast	20 mg PO twice daily
Zileuton	600 mg PO 4 times daily

5. *Beta$_2$ agonists*

Salbutamol	2–4 mg PO 2–3 times daily
Terbutaline	2 mg PO 2–3 times daily
Bambuterol	10 mg PO at bed time

6. *Phosphodiesterase inhibitors*

Theophylline	200–300 mg tab, SR, one tablet twice daily.
Aminophylline	5 mg/kg IV in 25% 20 ml dextrose

Inhalational steroids are the seat anchor of treatment in bronchial asthma which is an immunoinflammatory disease. Bronchodilators are only useful during exacerbation.

ACUTE BRONCHITIS

Essentials of diagnosis

- Fever, myalgia, headache, malaise.
- Dry cough initially – then with mucoid scanty expectoration.
- Prolonged expiration, scattered wheeze and fine crepitations.
- Mostly of viral etiology.

Treatment

- Steam inhalation.
- Antibiotics as prophylaxis against bacterial invasion, e.g. cephadroxyl 500 mg bid or quinolones for 3–5 days.
- Analgesics – antipyretics.

CHRONIC BRONCHITIS

Essentials of diagnosis

- Long history of productive cough with intermittent aggravation remission and productive cough lasting for 3 months or more for consecutive 2 years.
- Shortness of breath, cyanosis (blue bloaters)
- Scattered rhonchi and basal coarse crepitations.
- Dirty lung with increased bronchovascular markings in x-ray.

- Features of pulmonary hypertension clinically and in ECG.
- Increased Hb, reduced P_aO_2 and ↑ $PaCO_2$ in ABG.
- For differentiation from emphysema see Table 4.3.

Table 4.3: Differentiation of chronic bronchitis from emphysema

	Pink puffer (predominant emphysema)	Blue bloater (predominant bronchtis)
Clinical features:		
Onset	Dyspnoea and cough	Cough without dyspnoea
Build	Thin	Obese
Sputum	Scanty	Profuse, mucopurulent
Dyspnoea	Intesne with purse lip breathing	Relatively mild dyspnoea
Cough	After dyspnoea starts	Before dyspnoea starts
Cardiac failure	Rarely develop oedema or overt	Often oedematous and easily lapse
(Corpulmonale)	heart failure	into CHF
weight loss	Marked weight loss	No marked weight loss except terminally
Bronchial infections	Less frequent	More frequent
Episodes of res. failure	Often terminal	Repeated
Pulmonary hypertension	None or mild	Moderate to severe
Course	Unrelenting downhill	Ambulatory
Investigations:		
X-ray chest	Narrow cardiac shadow *Attenuated vessels* *Emphysema* Bullous changes	*Increased broncho- vascular markings*
Arterial Pa CO_2	Normal	Raised
Elastic recoil	Marked decrease	Normal
Resistance	Normal or slight increase	High
Diffusing capacity	Decreased	Normal

Treatment

- Since the disease is polymicrobial each episode of infective sputum be treated with cephadroxyl 500 mg bid, or quinolones or amoxycillin 500 mg tid for 5 days.
- Stop cigarette smoking.
- Inhalational β_2 agonists during exacerbation and ipratropium bromide as long term therapy.
- Oral theophylline, sustained release/time released form at bed time.
- Concentrated O_2 or CPAP if there is progressive hypoxemia and chronic respiratory failure.
- Short course of steroids – prednisolone 0.5 mg/kg/day for 14–21 days in advanced disease.
- Those with severe COPD may benefit form intermittent negative pressure ventilation or bilateral transnasal ventilation.

BRONCHIECTASIS

Essentials of diagnosis

- Profuse, purulent and putrid expectoration of long duration.
- Haemoptysis, recurrent pneumonia, clubbing, weight loss.
- Basal coarse crepitations, obstructive pulmonary dysfunction, honey combing in x-ray chest, crowded bronchial markings.
- CT scan and bronchography (only indicated if surgery contemplated).

Treatment

- Antibiotics based on sputum culture and sensitivity for 2–4 weeks.
- Chest physiotherapy with postural drainage
- In haled β_2 agonists for bronchodilatation

- Surgery is indicated for localised bronchiectasis not responding to medical treatment and for control of massive haemoptysis.

PNEUMONIA

Essentials of diagnosis

- Fever, cough, chest pain, dyspnoea; often hypothermia
- Bronchial (tubular) breath sounds.
- Airspace pneumonia or parenchymal infiltrate in x-ray chest respecting lobar boundaries.
- Severe physical symptoms but minimal chest signs in mycoplasma pneumonia
- Bulging fissures with predilection for upper lobes and red currant jelly sputum in Klebsiella pneumonia.
- Multiple pneumatoceles in staphylococcal pneumonia
- Cavitation is common in pseudomonas, staphylococcal, anaerobes and klebsiella pneumonia and empyema can complicate most forms except for pseudomonas infection.
- Pneumocystis pneumonia is often bilateral with ground glass appearance, ARDS, pneumothorax and respiratory failure – common to AIDS and immuno suppressed.
- Alcohol abuse, diabetes mellitus predispose to klebsiella pneumonia; cystic fibrosis and bronchiectasis to pseudomonas pneumonia and poor dental hygiene to pneumonia by anaerobes.

Treatment

- Penicillin, amoxycillin preferred for pneumococcal pneumonia.
- Cefotaxime, cefuroxime, ceftriaxone preferred for *H. influenzae* pneumonia.
- Cloxacillin with rifampicin or gentamicin preferred for staphylococcal pneumonia.

- Third generation cephalosporin plus aminoglycoside preferred for klebsiella pneumonia.
- Carbenicillin plus aminoglycoside for pseudomonas pneumonia.
- Amoxycillin – clavulanate (875 mg) tid or clindamycin 300–600 mg IV PO 6 hrly followed by penicillin + metronidazole for mixed infection.
- Doxycycline/erythromycin/azithromycin for myco-plasma pneumonia.
- Macrolide with rifampicin for legionella pneumonia.
- Doxycycline/azithromycin/quinolone for chlamydia – pneumonia.
- TMP-SMX or pentamide isoethionate plus prednisolone or clindamycin + primaquine or trimetrexate + folinic acid for pneumocystis pneumonia.

PULMONARY TUBERCULOSIS

Essentials of diagnosis

- Can be primary complex (in children) or reinfection (reactivation), see Table 4.4.
- Fatigue, lowgrade fever, weight loss, sweating and cough.
- Haemoptysis (Table 4.5) positive Mantoux test.

Table 4.4: Diferentiation of reinfection from primary complex

Reinfection	Primary complex
1. Absence of enlarged hilar lymph nodes	1. Enlargement of hilar lymph nodes
2. Usually subapical location	2. Any part of lung
3. Tendency to cavitation and progress	3. Usually heals, cavitation rare, thin-walled
4. Spread bronchogenic, hence disease is localised to the lungs	4. Spread by lymphatic route and hematogenous Miliary spread common
5. Healing of the lesion by fibrosis	5. Healing of lesion mainly by calcification

Table 4.5: Differences between haemoptysis and haematemesis

Haemoptysis	Haematemesis
1. Cough preceds haemoptysis	Nausea and vomiting precede haemetemesis
2. Frothy due to admixture of air	Not frothy
3. pH alkaline	pH acidic
4. Mixed with macrophage and neutrophil	Mixed with food particles
5. Malena absent	Malena present
6. Bright red in colour	Dark brown in colour due to acid haematin
7. Previous history of respiratory disease	Previous history of peptic ulcer disease
8. Diagnosed by bronchoscopy	Diagnosed by gastroscopy

- Pulmonary infiltrate, mostly apical, often with cavitation and mediastinal lymphadenopathy.
- Acid fast bacilli in sputum, positive sputum culture.
- Exclude diabetes mellitus, silicosis and HIV if disease is chronic or drug resistant.
- Mantoux is termed positive if (1) more than 5 mm in HIV positive, on immuno suppressants or lympho-proliferative disorder; (2) more than 15 mm in any person without risk factors for tuberculosis.

Treatment

- Rifampicin 10 mg/kg (mxm 600 mg) + INH 5 mg/kg (mxm 300 mg) + Ethambutol 15 mg/kg + Pyrazinamide 25 mg/kg; all in empty stomach for 2 months followed by rifampicin 10 mg/kg + INH 5 mg/kg daily for 4 months.
- Directly observed therapy (DOT) for all patients of resistant tuberculosis or those receiving twice weekly or thrice weekly regimes.
- Intermittent therapy can be in the form of (1) thrice a week rifampicin + INH + pyrazinamide + ethambutol/ streptomycin for 6 months; (2) initial daily above 4 drug therapy for 2 weeks followed by twice/thrice week 4 drug

therapy for 4 week followed by INH + rifampicin twice weekly for 4 months; (3) daily 4 drugs for 2 months followed by INH + rifampicin twice/thrice weekly for 4 months.

- In twice/thrice week regimes dose of antitubercular drugs is
  INH – 15 mg/kg (mxm 900 mg)
  Rifampicin 10 mg/kg (mxm 600 mg)
  Ethambutol – 25–50 mg/kg (mxm 2500 mg)
  Pyrazinamide 50–75 mg/kg (mxm 3 gm)
  Streptomycin 25–50 mg/kg (mxm 1.5 gm)
- Pyrazinamide is contraindicated in pregnant women,
- Pyridoxin 25–50 mg daily be given with INH to reduce CNS and peripheral nervous system side effects
- Multidrug resistant tuberculosis patients need 5 antitubercular drugs including cycloserine, azithromycin and quinolones for 12–24 months.
- Treatment of nontuberculous mycobacterial disease is

M. kansasii	Rifampicin + INH + ethambutol for 12–18 months
M. chelonei *M. fortuitum*	Amikacin + Qinolones + clarithromycin
M. avium intracellulare	Rifabutin + azithromycin + ethambutol.

- Non-healing tuberculous cavities may require thoracoplasty, laser therapy.

BRONCHOGENIC CARCINOMA

Essentials of diagnosis

- Anorexia, weight loss, chronic cough, haemoptysis, nonspecific chest pain, clubbing.

- Paraneoplastic syndrome — Horner's syndrome, SIADH, hypercalcemia, Eaton-Lambert myasthenia.
- Diagnosis is by CT scan/fiberoptic bronchoscopic biopsy/ fluorescent bronchoscopy/endobronchial ultrasound. Sputum cytology is highly specific but insensitive.

Treatment

Non small cell carcinoma

Stage I and stage II	Surgical resection
Stage IIIA	Resection + radiotherapy
Stage IIIB	Chemo-radiotherapy
StageIV	Need based paliation

Clinical features that preclude complete resection include involvement of pericardium, pleura, great vessels, esophagus, recurrent laryngeal nerve, trachea, carina, contralateral mediastinal nodes.

Small cell lung cancer

Chemotherapy with cisplatin plus etoposide along with radiation.

INTERSTITIAL LUNG DISEASE

Essentials of diagnosis

- Insidious dry cough, exertional dyspnoea, clubbing
- Late diffuse fine inspiratory crackles
- Restrictive ventilatory deficit and reducing diffusing capacity
- Positive ANA, RF; transbronchial biopsy diagnostic

Treatment

Longterm lowdose corticosteroids
Interferon gamma Ib.

PULMONARY EOSINOPHILIA

Essentials of diagnosis

- Dry cough, especially at night often with wheezing, dyspnoea
- High blood eosinophilia with usually peripheral infiltrates
- PFT shows mild restrictive defect.
- Can be due to chronic eosinophilic pneumonia (a disease of women), drugs (nitrofurantoin, phenytoin, ranitidine) helminths (filarial worms, strongyloids, ankylostomiasis), Churg-Strauss syndrome, primary pulmonary histoplasmosis, aspergillosis, etc.

Table 4.6: Topical eosinophilia vs bronchial asthma

	Bronchial asthma	Tropical eosinophilia
History	Usually starts	Any age
Age	before 3 years of age	
Duration of	Long duration	Short duration
symptoms		
Cough and	Paroxymal cough	Dyspnoea more than
Dyspnoea	more than	cough
	dyspnoea	Breathlessness
		particularly after
		bout of cough
Fever	Rare	Common
Loss of weight	Seldom	Fairly common
Auscultatory		
Signs:	Compatible with	Disproportion
	degree of cough	between cough and
	and breathlessness	breathlessness and signs
Investigations:		
Blood	Normal WBC count	Leucocytosis,
	Eosinophils 8–15%.	eosinophilia marked
X-ray	Increased bronchial	Mottling may be
	markings	seen
Treatment	No known cure	Diethylcarbamazine
		specific

Treatment

- For filarial disease (Loeffler syndrome) – diethyl carbamazine 5 mg/kg/day in 3 divided doses for 14–21 days.
- For chronic eosinophilic pneumonia – prednisolone i mg/kg/day for 10 days with tapering and maintenance dose for 1 year
- For no apparent extrinsic cause short term corticosteroid in above dosage. Response to steroid is dramatic but recurrences are common.

PULMONARY EMBOLISM

Essentials of diagnosis

- Dyspnoea, chest pain, haemoptysis, syncope, mimicking acute mI (Table 4.7).
- Tachypnoea, wide A-a PO_2.
- Predisposition to venous thrombosis, usually of lower extremity.
- Features of pulmonary hypertension, RV strain.
- Increased plasma and urinary D.dimer.
- Characteristic defect in V/Q scan, spiral CT and pulmonary angiography.

Treatment

- Anticoagulation with heparin or low molecular weight heparin followed by oral anticoagulants for 6 months. This reduces chances of reembolism and facilitates natural clot dissolution (secondary prevention)
- Thrombolytic therapy – with tPA if patient remains haemodynamically instable despite heparin therapy
- Trans jugular venacaval filter placement when thromboembolism is recurrent.
- Supportive treatment with rest, oxygen inhalation, antibiotic.

Table 4.7: Differentiation of massive pulmonary embolism from myocardial infarction

	Pulmonary embolism	*Myocardial infarction*
History	Convalescent	Of angina of effort
Pain	Severe, usually central chest pain	Pressing or crushing substernal radiating to shoulder or arm
Shock	Frequently first symptom	Usually after several hours of increasing pain
Gallop	Adjacent to sternum, increased by insp.	Apical, louder during exp.
Cough	Severe	Rare
Cyanosis	May be marked	Mild or none
Hemaptysis	May occur later	None
Fever	Early, may reach high level	24–36 hours after onset, moderate
JVP	Raised	Normal
Heart sounds	Loud pulmonary 2nd sound and systolic murmur	Feeble heart sounds or gallop rhythm
X-ray	Pulmonary infarction	Not characteristic
ECG	Right axis deviation, right artial P waves, RBBB.	Typical according to location of infarction

PULMONARY HYPERTENSION

Essentials of diagnosis

- Dyspnoea, chest pain, exertional syncope.
- Narrow split S_2 with loud P_2, RVH..
- Enlarged MPA in chest x-ray; ECG evidence of RVH and RA enlargement.
- Hypoxemia and increased wasted ventilation in PFT.

Treatment

- Treatment of inciting factor like R-L shunt, recurrent thromboembolism, etc.
- Pulmonary vasodilators, e.g. calcium channel blockers, prostacycline infusion, endothelin antagonist

(bosentan), nitric oxide inhalation, sildenafil, etc. may help in mild to moderate disease.
- Heart lung transplantation in advanced cases.
- Control of heart failure if present.

COR PULMONALE

Essentials of diagnosis

- Symptoms and signs of chronic bronchitis and emphysema.
- ↑ JVP, ascites, hepatomegaly, edema.
- P pulmonale, right axis deviation and RVH in ECG.
- Enlarged PA and RV in chest x-ray.

Treatment

- Treatment of inciting pulmonary disease like chronic bronchitis and emphysema.
- Control of RVF with diuretics, salt and fluid restriction (digoxin has no role in right heart failure unless atrial fibrillation is present).
- Oxygen inhalation.
- Treatment of chronic pulmonary insufficiency with CPAP, enriched oxygen and bronchodilators.

BRONCHOPULMONARY ASPERGILLOSIS

Essentials of diagnosis

- Features of bronchial asthma with peripheral high eosinophilia.
- Pulmonary infiltrates (transient or fixed).
- Central bronchiectasis, raised IgE.
- Precipitating antibodies to aspergillus antigen so also positive skin testing.

Treatment

- Prednisolone 1 mg/kg/day for 2 months with gradual tapering.
- Itraconazole 200 mg daily or twice daily, when response to steroid is short-lived.
- Bronchodilators.

HYPERSENSITIVE PNEUMONITIS

Essentials of diagnosis

- Sudden onset of malaise, chill, fever, cough, dypnoea on exposure to responsible antigen.
- Bibasilar crackles, tachypnoea, tachycardia (no rhonchi)
- Small bilateral nodular densities sparing apex and bases.
- Restrictive dysfunction in PFT, with ↓ diffusing capacity.

Treatment

- Avoidance of exposure to offending agent.
- Prednisolone 0.5 mg/kg daily, tapered over 4–6 weeks.

PLEURAL EFFUSION

Essentials of diagnosis

- Chest pain, lethargy, mild fever; but can be asymptomatic; dyspnoea in large effusion.
- Dullness on percussion, decreased breath sounds over effusion; bronchial breath sounds and aegophony above effusion.
- Radiographic evidence of effusion, with passive collapse (Tables 4.8, 4.9).
- Pleural fluid samples show increased protein, diminished glucose and rise in LDH in exudative effusion.

Table 4.8: Differentiation between active and passive collapse

Features	Active collapse	Passive collapse
Droop of shoulder; hollowing of supra and infra clavicular fossa	Present	Absent
Trachea	Pulled to same side	Pushed to opposite side
Percussion note	Dull	Subtympanitic or skodiac resonance
Breath sounds	Absent	Tubular
VF/VR	Absent	Increased
Cause	Luminal or extraluminal obstruction	Pleural effusion Pneumothorax

Table 4.9: Differentiation between fibrosis and collapse

Features	Fibrosis	Collapse
1. Onset	Chronic	Sudden
2. Clubbing	Present	Absent
3. Percussion	Impaired	Dull
4. Breath sounds	Decreased	Absent
5. Added sounds	Crackles	None

Treatment

- Transudative effusion occurs in absence of pleural disease (nephrosis, cirrhosis, CHF, myxedema) and regresses with treatment of primary disease.
- In exudative effusion tuberculosis is the most common and needs 6–9 months of ATT with short course of steroid to reduce pleural fibrosis.
- Parapneumonic uncomplicated effusions resolve completely with antibiotic treatment of pneumonia.
- Malignant pleural effusion commonly accompanying carcinoma breast and bronchus is treated with repeated thoracentesis or tube placement. Pleurodesis with talc or doxycycline instillation may be required.

- After resolution of effusion patient be advised deep breathing exercises to bring about expansion of the lung.

EMPYEMA

Essentials of diagnosis

- Fever, toxaemia, chill; bulging intercostal spaces.
- Thick exudative pleural fluid, positive Gram stain and culture.
- Concurrent pneumonia or tubercular effusion.
- Pleural fluid pH < 7.2 with very low glucose, high LDH and abundant poly morphs.

Treatment

- Antibiotics as per culture-sensitivity; ATT for preceding tubercular effusion.
- Tube drainage; intrapleural fibrinolytic agents – (urokinase/streptokinase) to facilitate drainage.
- Thoracoplasty/muscle flap when empyema cavity refuses to heal.

PNEUMOTHORAX

Essentials of diagnosis

- Acute onset of chest pain and dyspnoea.
- Hyper resonance, diminished breath sounds (Tables 4.10, 4.11).
- Mediastinal shift, cyanosis and hypotension in tension pneumothorax.
- X-ray shows pleural air and mediastinal shift, collapsed lung.

Treatment

- Small and stable pneumothorax (<15% of hemithorax) resolve spontaneously but O_2 supplement may increase clearance.

- For large or progressive pneumothorax – tube drainage with one way Heimlich valve.
- Tension pneumothorax or very large pneumothorax – tube thoracostomy with underwater seal drainage.

Table 4.10: Differential diagnosis of common types of pneumothorax

Spontaneous pneumothorax	Tuberculous pneumothorax
No family history of tuberculosis	Family history of tuberculosis may be obtained
Fever usually absent	Pyrexia common
No loss of weight	Weight loss common
No sweats	Night sweats frequent
Other lung normal	Other lung may show signs of tubercle
Fluid accumulation minimal or absent	Fair amount of fluid may accumulate
No adhesions present	Adhesions frequently

Table 4.11: Causes of resonant note with diminished breath sounds

Pneumothorax	Large pulmonary cavity
1. Acute onset	1. Insidious onset.
2. Chest pain.	2. No chest pain
3. Absence of movements of chest on affected side.	3. Restriction of movement at apex only
4. Bulging of interspaces VR diminished or absent. Breath sounds absent	4. Retraction of interspaces Increased VR Cavernous or amphoric breath sounds
Cracked pot sound rare. cavity superficial Succussion splash may be present Bell tympany constant.	Cracked pot sound usually if No succussion splash Bell tympany rare.

OBESITY–HYPOVENTILATION SYNDROME

Essentials of diagnosis

- Loud cyclical snoring, breath cessation, thrashing limb movements during sleep
- Day time somnolence/fatigue/headache, cognitive impairment
- Short neck, narrow oropharynx
- Polysomnography reveals apneic episodes, fall in P_aO_2 and arrhythmias

Treatment

- Weight reduction, avoidance of alcohol
- Nasal CPAP
- Uvulopaltopharyngoplasty with laser eliminates snoring more than apnoea.

ACUTE RESPIRATORY DISTRESS SYNDROME

Essentials of diagnosis

- Acute onset of respiratory failure ($P_aO_2 < 60$ mm Hg, $P_aCO_2 > 50$ mm Hg).
- Bilateral radiographic pulmonary infiltrate, ground glass appearance.
- Normal LA pressure and PAWP (< 18 mm Hg).
- P_aO_2 to $FIO_2 < 200$, regardless the level of PEEP.

Treatment

- Treatment of preciipitating cause and sepsis if any
- PEEP and supplemental O_2 to keep P_aO_2 above 60 mmHg and SaO_2 above 90%.
- Prone positioning.
- Depamine infusion if PEEP causes fall in cardiac output.

EMPHYSEMA

Essentials of diagnosis

- Dyspnoea, poor exercise tolerance, tympanic percussion note, decreased breath sounds (Table 4.12).
- Obliteration of liver, and cardiac dullness.
- X-ray evidence of hyperinflation, parenchymatous bulla, subpleural bleb.
- $\downarrow P_aO_2$ but normal P_aCO_2.

Treatment

- Human- alpha$_1$ antitrypsin 60 mg/kg IV weekly in alpha$_1$ antitrypsin deficiency.
- Reduction pneumoplasty, bullectomy
- Supportive therapy with supplemental O_2, CPAP, and often lung transplantation.

Table 4.12: Differentiating features between emphysema and chronic bronchitis

Features	Predominant emphysema (pink puffer)	Predominant bronchitis (blue bloater)
1. Age of onset	6th decade	5th decade
2. Cough	After dyspnoea	Before dyspnoea
3. Dyspnoea	Severe	Mild
4. Sputum	Scanty, mucoid	Copious, purulent
5. Infections	Less common	Common
6. Respiratory insufficiency	Often terminal	Repeated attacks
7. Chest X-ray	Hyperinflation Bullous changes; Small heart	Increased broncho-vascular markings; Large heart
8. PaCO$_2$ (mm Hg)	35–40	50–60
PaO$_2$ (mm Hg)	65–75	45–60
9. Pulmonary hypertension	Mild	Moderate to severe
10. C or poulmonale	Preterminal stage	Common
11. Diffusing capacity	Decreased	Normal to slight reduction

5

CARDIOVASCULAR DISEASES

CONGESTIVE HEART FAILURE

Essentials of diagnosis

- Left ventricular failure – Exertional dyspnoea, cough, fatigue, orthopnea, paroxysmal nocturnal dyspnoea, gallop rhythm.
- Right ventricular failure – raised JVP, tender hepatomegaly, dependent edema
- S_3, cardiomegaly, basal crepitations
- Associated findings – anemia, thyromegaly, valvular stenosis/regurgitation, myocarditis, evidence of pulmonary hypertension.
- ↑ arm to tongue circulation time, ↑ 'B' ANP, dilated atria and ventricles with poor EF,
- Pulmonary venous hypertension, interstitial edema in chest x-ray.

Treatment

- Salt restricted diet, decreased physical activity.
- ACE inhibitors – usually in combination with a diuretic are the drugs of first choice (reduce mortality by 20%); alternatively angiotensin II receptor blocker (losartan, valsetran) can be given – addition of spironolactone may be beneficial but hyperkalemia be avoided.
- Low dose betablocker (carvedilol 3.125 mg bid/bisoprolol 1.25 mg, metoprolol 12.5 mg) may be tried.
- Digoxin 0.125 – 0.25 mg orally 5 days a week as maintenance; loading dose of 0.75–1.25 mg over 24–48 hours may be given if early effect is desired. Safe plasma

level of digoxin is 0.7–1.2 ng/ml. Role of digoxin in patients of CHF with sinus rhythm is limited.

- Vasodilators – isosorbide dinitrate 20–80 mg tid or IV nitroglycerine/nitropruside for acute cases. Nesiretide, recombinant human brain natriuretic peptide, 2 µg/kg IV bolus, then 0.01 µg/kg/min infusion is also a good vasodilator. Hydralazine 25 mg tid orally is also effective but because of techycardia and hypotension is replaced by angiotensin receptor blocker.
- Other inotropic agents – like milrinone or dobutamine when other measures fail.
- Anticoagulation if ejection fraction is poor particularly those with recent MI or have atrial fibrillation
- Biventricular pacing (RV apex and LV lateral wall through coronary sinus) improves EF as in an CHF patients there is abnormal intraventricular conduction
- Implantable ventricular assist device, cardiomyoplasty, LV reduction surgery are only bridge to cardiac transplantation in very advanced cases.

ACUTE PULMONARY EDEMA

Essentials of diagnosis

- Dyspnoea, cyanosis, tachycardia, diaphoresis, pink frothy sputum.
- Fine crepitation, rhonchi and expiratory wheeze.
- S_3 gallop
- Chest x-ray shows interstitial and alveolar edema (butterfly pattern).
- Arterial hypoxemia, raised pulmonary capillary wedge pressure in cardiogenic pulmonary edema.

Treatment

- Sitting position with legs dangling over bed side.
- O_2 inhalation/noninvasive pressure support ventilation.

- Morphine 4–8 mg IV, repeated every 2–4 hours.
- IV furosemide 40 mg or bumentanide 1 mg.
- Oral/IV vasodilator therapy (see under CHF).
- IV aminophylline 5 mg/kg or inhaled betadrenergic agonists.

MYOCARDITIS

Essentials of diagnosis

- Chest pain (pleuritic/non-pleuritic), often following upper respiratory infection.
- ECG shows tachycardia, non specific repolarisation changes, arrhythmias, intraventricular conduction anomalies.
- Evidence of CHF, gallop rhythm, cardiomegaly and contractile dysfunction.
- Myocardial biopsy diagnostic, else gallium 67 scintigraphy.

Treatment

- Specific antimicrobial therapy if infective agent identified.
- Azathioprine plus prednisolone if immunologic mechanism suspected but good outcome cannot be predicted.
- Treatment of heart failure and arrhythmias (digoxin is not indicated).
- Spontaneous improvement may occur but many degenerate to dilated cardiomyopathy.

DILATED CARDIOMYOPATHY

Essentials of diagnosis

- Symptoms and signs of heart failure with functional TR, S_3 gallop.

- Low QRS voltage in ECG, nonspecific repolarisation abnormalities, intraventricular conduction abnormalities.
- Cardiac dilatation in x-ray; poor LV function in Echo.

Treatment

- Abstinence from alcohol; treatment of thyroid dysfunction.
- Management of congestive failure (digoxin low dose may help but dobutamine/dopamine are beneficial).
- Long term anticoagulation.
- Dual chamber pacing may help but cardiac transplant is often required.

HYPERTROPHIC CARDIOMYOPATHY

Essentials of diagnosis

- Chest pain, dyspnoea, syncope, similar symptom in family members.
- Sustained apical impulse, S_4, systolic ejection murmur increased by valsalva (Table 5.1).

Table 5.1: Differential diagnosis of systolic murmurs

Clinical signs	HOCM	Aortic valvar stenosis
Double apex impulse	Common	Less common
Presystolic gallop	Common	Less common
Single 2nd sound	Less common	Common
Paradoxical splitting of 2nd sound	Common	Less common
Systolic thrill	Not common	Common
Systolic murmur	Along left sternal border and at apex	2nd right inter space radiating to neck
Diastolic murmur or AR	Rare	Common
Carotid pulse	Visible, rapid upstroke	Invisible, slow upstroke
Valsalva manoeuvre	Murmur louder	Murmur softer

- ECG – LVH, Septal Q waves prominent.
- Echo – asymmetric LV hypertrophy, SAM of mitral valve, hypercontractile LV with diastolic dysfunction.

Treatment

- Betablocker or verapamil.
- Septal ablation by alcohol injection to involved branch from LCA.
- Dual chamber pacing may delay progress of hypertrophy and obstruction.

RESTRICTIVE CARDIOMYOPATHY

Essentials of diagnosis

- Dyspnoea, effort intolerance, features of CHF, Kussmaul's sign.
- ECG – low voltage, conduction anomalies, ST-T changes
- Normal to mildly reduced LV function, square root sign in cardiac cath; mimics constrictive pericarditis (Table 5.2).

Table 5.2: Differentiating features of constrictive pericarditis and restrictive cardiomyopathy

Features	Constrictive pericarditis	Restrictive cardiomyopathy
1. Symptoms	Of underlying disease	Of underlying disease
2. JVP		
a. Prominent 'y' descent	Present	Absent
b. Prominent 'x' descent	Absent	Present
c. Kussmaul's sign	Present	Present or absent
3. S_3	Absent	Absent
4. Pericardial knock	Present	Absent
5. ECG Low voltage complexes	May be present	May be present

Features	Constrictive pericarditis	Restrictive cardiomyopathy
6. Echocardiography		
a. Thickened pericardium	Present	Absent
b) RV size	Usually normal	Usually normal
c) Myocardial thickness	Normal	Usually increased
7. Cardiac catheterisation		
a) RA/LA pressure	Equal	LA>RA
b) Variation of RA pressure with respiration	Absent	Present
c) Ventricular diastolic pressures	Equal in RV & LV	LV > RV by more than 5 mm Hg.
d) PCWP	< 18 mm Hg.	> 18 mm Hg.
e) Pulmonary artery pressure	< 50 mm Hg.	> 50 mm Hg.
8. Biopsy of myocardium	Not helpful	May be helpful

Treatment

• Diuretics in low dosage and steroids but outcome is usually poor.

ACUTE RHEUMATIC FEVER

Essentials of diagnosis

• Evidence of carditis (tachycardia, heart failure, mitral regurgitation PR prolongation); subcutaneous nodules, erythema marginatum, fleeting polyarthritis or polyarthralgia, Sydenham's chorea (least common but most diagnostic).
• Age group 5–15 years, fever, raised ESR and CRP.
• Positive streptococcal antibodies titers (antistreptolysin 'O' and anti DNAase B).

- Unexplained CHF or mitral systolic murmur/MVP is a child demands exclusion of ARF.

Treatment

- Strict bed rest till fever, tachycardia, ESR and ECG (PR interval) return to normal.
- Aspirin – 50 mg/kg upto 3 gram in 4–6 divided dose.
- Procaine penicillin 6 lac units IM daily for 10 days.
- Prednisolone 1 mg/kg with tapering over 2 weeks when carditis is prominent.
- Inj. benzathine penicillin 1.2 MU IM 3 weekly for 5 years or upto age of 25 years to prevent recurrence.

PERICARDIAL EFFUSION

- Chest pain, cough, dyspnoea (in tamponade).
- Pericardial friction rub, large heart in x-ray chest.
- In tamponade – tachycardia, tachypnoea, narrow pulse pressure, pulsus paradoxus, raised JVP, ascites.
- ECG – low QRS voltage, nonspecific ST, T changes; Echo – diagnostic.
- Small effusion need observation; for tamponade pericardiocentesis followed by complete catheter drainage.
- Partial pericardiectomy (thoracoscopic) if effusion recurrent or due to malignancy/uraemia.
- Treatment of primary cause, e.g. tuberculosis, neoplastic disease, hypothyroidism, etc.
- In constrictive pericarditis ascites, edema, hepatic congestion, raised JVP, positive Kussmaul's sign are evident but pulsus paradoxus is rare.
- Heart size may be normal, pericardial calcification is evident and echo/CT show pericardial thickening.
- Treatment is with diuretics followed by pericardiectomy.

SYSTEMIC HYPERTENSION

Essentials of diagnosis

- Mild to moderate hypertension is asymptomatic; any type of headache may accompany but suboccipital pulsating headache in early morning is characteristic.
- Accelerated hypertension is associated with confusion, visual disturbances, somnolence and vomiting (hypertensive encephalopathy).
- Exertional and often paroxysmal nocturnal dyspnoea may occur (LV dysfunction); coronary artery disease often associated.
- Cerebral involvement can cause stroke due to thrombosis, haemorrhage.
- Associated features of inciting event, i.e. pheochromo-cytoma, Con's syndrome, hyperthyroidism, coarctation, nephritis.
- Blood pressure persistently above 140/90 mm Hg on recording at 3 occassions.
- Documentation of LV hypertrophy, diastolic dysfunction, retinopathy, renal disease, etc.
- Exclusion of spurious rise in BP as in elderly in presence of Osler's sign, i.e. palpable brachial or radial artery when the cuff is inflated above systolic pressure.

Treatment

a. *Nonpharmacologic therapy:* Smoking cessation, weight reduction if obese, limitation of alcohol intake to 60 ml/d, aerobic exercise, reduction in salt intake, diet rich in fruits, vegetables and low in total and saturated fat, adequate calcium, potassium and magnesium, meditation and yoga.

b. *Drug Therapy*

1. *Diuretics:* Hydrochlorthiazide 25 mg once daily; chlorthalidone 25 mg once daily; indapamide 2.5–5 mg daily; bumetanide – 0.25 mg daily; torsemide 2.5 mg

daily or combination like hydrochlorthiazide + amiloride 5 mg/spironolactone 25 mg/triamterine – 50 mg.

2. *Betablockers:* Aetinol 25–200 mg daily, betaxolol 10– 40 mg daily, cartelol 2.5–10 mg daily, carvedilol 6.25 to 100 mg in two divided doses daily, nadolol 20–160 mg daily, pindolol 10–60 mg in two divided doses, propranolol 40–320 mg in two divided doses, timolol 10–40 mg in 2 doses, metoprolol 50–200 mg daily.

3. *ACE inhibitors:* Benzapril 10 mg daily, captopril 25 mg twice daily, enalapril 5–10 mg daily, fosinopril 10 mg daily; lisinopril 5–10 mg daily, moexipril 7.5–30 mg daily; perindopril 4–16 mg daily; quinapril 10–80 daily; ramipril 2.5–20 mg daily, trandolapril 1–8 mg daily.

4. *Angiotensin II receptor blockers:* Candesetral 16–32 mg daily;eprosartan 600 mg daily; irbesartan 150–300 mg daily; losartan 50–100 mg daily, telmisartan 40– 80 mg daily, valsartan 80–320 mg daily.

5. *Calcium channel blockers:* Nifedipine 30–120 mg/d, amlodipine 5–20 mg/d, felodipine 5–20 mg/d, isradipine 2.5–5 mg/d, nislodipine 20–60 mg/d, verapamil 120– 480 mg/d, diltiazem 180–360 mg in two doses.

6. *Alfa adrenoceptor blocking agent:* Prazosin 2–20 mg in 2–3 doses, terazosin 1–20 mg in 2 divided doses, doxazosin 1–16 mg/d

7. *Sympatholytics / methyl dopa:* 500–2000 mg/d in two doses; guanfacine 1–3 mg qd, guanabenz 8–64 mg in two doses, clonidine 0.2–0.6 mg in 2 doses/patch/TTS weekly.

8. *Peripheral neuronal antagonists:* Guanethidine 10– 100 mg qd, guanadrel 5 mg bid, reserpine 0.05–0.25 mg qd.

9. *Direct vasodilators:* Hydralazine 50–300 mg in 2–4 divided doses, minoxidil – 5–40 mg qd.

Selection of antihypertensive regimen depends not only the degree of elevated blood pressure but age, renal status, associated comorbid condition. ACE inhibitors are preferred in diabetes, heart failure, post-myocardial infarction, isolated systolic hypertension, atherosclerotic vascular disease, Diuretics are effective in all ages but more so for isolated systolic hypertension of the elderly. Betablockers are preferred for young, those with ischaemic heart disease, migraine, hyperthyroid state but be avoided in asthma, depression, diabetes mellitus, gout, heart block, heart failure, peripheral vascular disease. Commonly useful multidrug regimens are (1) a diuretic plus a betablockers plus a vasodilator or a calcium channel blocker; (2) diuretic plus an ACE inhibitor plus a sympatholytic or calcium channel blocker; (3) ACE inhibitor plus a calcium channel blocker plus betablocker or a sympatholytic.

Treatment of malignant hypertension

Systolic pressure above 220 mmHg or diastolic pressure above 125 mmHg, often with papilloedema. Hypertensive emergencies include encephalopathy (headache, confusion, irritability due to cerebrovascular spasm), nephropathy (hematuria, proteinuria), intracranial haemorrhage, aortic dissection, pulmonary edema. The goal is to reduce BP by no more than 25% within 1–2 hours and then to 160/100 mmHg within 2–6 hrs. Excessive reductions may precipitate coronary, cerebral and renal ischaemia.

1. IV agents — Nitroprusside is the agent of choice for most serious emergencies, dose is 0.25 – 10 µg/kg/min. Nitroglycerine 0.25–0.5 µg/kg/min is preferred in presence of myocardial ischaemia. Esmolol 500 µg/kg/min in 1 minute followed by 25–200 µg/kg/min is the alternative. Diazoxide 15–30 mg/min IV infusion or trimethaphan 0.5–5 mg/min infusion are equally effective. Labetalol 20–40 mg every 10 minutes or 2 mg/min infusion; enalaprilat 1.25 mg every 6 hours,

hydralazine 5–20 mg IV every 20 minutes,. furosemide 10–80 mg IV can also be used.

2. Oral agents — Nifedipine 10 mg SL, clonidine 0.1 mg every hour upto 8 doses, fenoldopam 0.1 µg/kg are less dependable.

ANGINA PECTORIS

Essentials of diagnosis

- Retrosternal squeezing or pressure like pain lasting for less than 30 minutes; radiating to inner side of left arm, to left shoulder, neck, jaw and teeth (any dermatome from C_8 to T_4).
- Precipitated by exertion, emotion, sexual activity, cold wind, climbing up stairs but promptly relieved by rest / nitro glycerine.
- Some have no pain but angina equivalents like sudden dizziness, fatigue, dyspnoea.
- Examination during pain may reveal midsystolic murmur of papillary muscle dysfunction, S_3, S_4.
- Evidence of hypertension, hyperlipidemia, dysthyroid state, HOCM, aortic valve disease, diabetes mellitus, homocystinemia, etc.
- ECG may show ST depression, T inversion (25–50% have normal resting ECG).
- Treadmil stress test shows evidence of ischaemia in the leads corresponding to coronary anatomy.
- Stress thallium shows dyskinesia, akinesia, hypokinesia in the ischaemic segment.
- Dipyridamole/dobutamine stress echo yield similar result.
- Coronary angiography is of last resort.
- The anginal pain should be differentiated from intercostal neuritis, Teiz syndrome, cervical spondylosis, pleuritis, cervical rib, reflux esophagitis, motor disorders of esophagus, mitral valve prolapse (Table 5.3).

Table 5.3: Angina pectoris *vs* myocardial infarction

	Angina pectoris	Myocardial infarction
1. Exciting factor	After exertion, cold or heavy meals	Without visible cause. Usually during rest at night
2. Attitude	Immobile	Restless
3. Pain		
Site	Retrosternal	Usually retrosternal but may be precordial
Duration	Never more than 5 minutes	About ½ an hour or more
Radiation	To both arms, neck or jaw	Not so diffuse
Relief	Nitrites	Nitrites have no effect
4. Vomiting	Absent	Common
5. Dyspnoea	None.Only breath held	Common
6. Shock	Absent	Marked
7. Sweating	Slight	Profuse
8. Fever	Absent	Present
9. Heart sounds	Normal	Weak,gallop rhythm
10. Pericarditis	Normal	May occur
11. Pulse	Normal or rapid	Small, rapid. often irregular
12. B.P.	Normal or increased	Tendency to fall
13. Cardiac failure	Absent	Occurs early
14. Cardiac enzymes	Normal	Raised
15. ECG	Transitory change during attack	Progressive, typical changes

Treatment

- Sublingual nitroglycerine 0.3–0.6 mg, 1 tab/glyceryl trinitrate 0.5 mg or sublingual isosorbide dinitrate 10 mg during pain. Pain not responding to above drugs or lasting for more than 30 minutes implies myocardial infarction
- Isosorbide 5 mononitrate 10–20 mg twice daily or 30–60 mg sustained release 1 tab daily morning;

nocturnal angina taken care of by nitroglycerine 2% ointment, at bed time.

- Sustained release NTG 2.5 mg capsule and continuous release glyceryne trinitrate 2.6 mg tablet are also available for long-term effect.
- Aspirin 325 mg or colospirin 100 mg, ecospirin 75 mg, delispirin 150 mg daily for antiplatelet effect, often with clopidogrel 75 mg daily or ticlopidine 250 mg twice daily.
- Betablockers – Atinolol 25–50 mg daily or metoprolol 50–100 mg daily to decrease myocardial contractility, can control increase of heart rate with emotion/exercise
- Trimetazidine 20 mg twice daily, oxyphedrine 4 mg qid, lidoflazine 60 mg daily have supportive role.
- Treatment of obesity, hypertension, diabetes hyperlipidemia, homocystinemia, etc.
- Endocardial protection with antioxidants, statins and ACE inhibitors.

UNSTABLE ANGINA

- Severe anginal pain; angina at rest with normal heart rate, new onset angina.
- Besides fixed obstruction, there is platelet thrombus, hence higher chances of being complicated by infarction.

Treatment

- Immediate hospitalization.
- Aspirin 325 mg, O_2 inhalation.
- IV nitroglycerine infusion.
- GP IIb/IIIA inhibitors IV, followed by balloon angioplasty.

VARIANT ANGINA

- Anginal pain unrelated to exertion, with ST elevation in ECG; pain and ECG changes can be provoked by IV ergonovine 0.05–4 mg.

* *Treatment* is with calcium channel blocker (verapamil 5 mg IV) or diltiazem orally, nifedipine 5 mg sublingual.

MYOCARDIAL INFARCTION

Essentials of diagnosis

* Retrosternal chest pain, squeezing or vice like, lasting for more than 30 minutes not relieved by rest, nitroglycerine; can mimic aortic dissection (Table 5.4).
* Nausea, vomiting, sweating, dizziness, fainting, syncope, hypotension, tachycardia, S_4, S_3 gallop, mitral regurgitation due to papillary muscle infarction, raised JVP, fine crepitation in lung fields.
* ECG — ST caving, inverted T waves, pathological Q waves.
* Raised troponin, CPK MB, CRP, SGOT, LDH.
* 2D echo shows the dyskinetic – hypokinetic infarcted segment, associated MR, LV clot.
* Hot spot scanning shows the infarcted region as "hot spots", indicated when ECG interpretation is difficult due to LBBB or CPK – MB rise is minimal.

Table 5.4: Myocardial infarction *vs* dissecting aortic aneurysm

	Dissecting aneurysm	*Myocardial infarction*
Fainting	Common	Uncommon
Pain	Chest or back, transmitted to both arms or legs	Precordial or epigastric, transmitted to left or back arm.
	Peak intensity at onset	Increases in intensity after it commences
Nervous symptoms	Possible paralysis	Nil
Murmur	Aortic diastolic murmur murmur may appear	Apical systolic may be heard
B.P.	Remains high	Falls
Other arteries	May show signs of involvement	Not affected

Treatment

- Hospitalization, absolute bed rest.
- Aspirin 325 mg, O_2 inhalation.
- Morphine 3 mg IV every 15 – 20 minutes for pain relief
- Thrombolytic therapy with Streptokinase 1.5 million units infused over I hr along with hydrocortisone, or urokinase 2.5 lac units IV over 2 minutes followed by 5 lac units over next 60 miniutes or rtPA 10 mg IV bolus, then 50 mg IV over 1 hr.
- Thrombolytic therapy is followed by SC heparin 5.000 units twice daily or LMW heparin for 5 days.
- *Management of complications*
  a. Sinus bradycardia especially associated with inferior wall MI responds to atropine
  b. Complete AV block of inferior wall MI responds to steroids, temporary pacing and isoprenaline/atropine
  c. Xylocaine infusion for VPB (> 6/minute) 1 mg/kg bolus followed by 2 mg/minute infusion
  d. IV propranolol 1–2 mg reduces chance of arrhythmia
- Oral rampiril/enlapril to limit infarct size and remodelling of myocardium.
- Gradual ambulation.
- Routine soft laxatives, light meals and adequate sleep
- IV Saline if there is RV infarction.
- Risk stratification by limited Treadmill after 3 weeks.
- Coronary angiography followed by ballooning with stenting or CABG as the case demands.

ARRHYTHMIAS

Paroxysmal Supraventricular Tachycardias (PSVT)

- Sudden palpitation, dizziness, syncope: patients can have angina and heart failure.
- ECG shows heart rate of 150 – 250/min, morphologically normal QRS complexes (Table 5.5).

- When PSVT causes angina or haemodynamic compromise immediate electrical cardioversion with 200–300 Joules is required.
- In non emergent cases try – carotid sinus massage one side at a time, valsalva, eye ball pressure, splashing of cold water to face.
- Pharmacologic conversion with IV adenosine 6 mg/ verapamil 5 mg/propranolol 1 mg/digoxin 0.5 mg/ esmolol 0.5 mg.
- Prevent recurrence by verapamil 40–80 mg daily or amiodarone 200–400 mg daily.
- If there is associated WPW syndrome, consider catheter RF ablation of bypass tract.

Table 5.5: Differential diagnosis of regular tachycardia

	Sinus tachycardia	Supraventricular tachycardia	Ventricular tachycardia	Atrial flutter with 2:1 block
1. Onset and termination	Gradual	Sudden	Sudden	May be sudden
2. Heart disease	Absent	Often absent	Usually present	Usually present
3. Heart rate	Rarely more than 160	160 or more	160 or more	Usually 150
4. Cannon waves	Absent	Regular cannon waves may be seen	Irregular cannon waves	Regular cannon waves
5. I st heart sound	Constant	Constant	Variable Intensity	Constant
6. Carotid sinus pressure	Gradual slowing with gradual return to previous rate on release of pressure	No change or abrupt reversion to normal	No change	Abrupt slowing for few beats only

TABLE 5.6: Differential diagnosis of irregular tachycardia

	Multiple ectopic beats	*A. fibrillation*	*A. flutter (with varying block)*
1. Associated condition	Idiopathic, Ischaemic heart disease, digitalis toxicity, etc.	Rheumatic heart disease, Thyrotoxicosis Ischaemic, or Hypertensive heart disease, or none	Same as in A. fibrillation
2. Rate at apex	Usually less than 120	More than 120	About 160
3. Effect of exercise	Disappear	Rhythm becomes more irregular	May become regular
4. Pulse apex deficit	May be present	Marked	None
5. Heart sounds	Occasionally only Ist sound heard	Vary in intensity	Variation of Ist heart sound
6. Other features	Long pauses preceded by premature beats Irregular cannon waves in jugular pulse	Pauses without preceding premature beats. More often permanent	Jugular pulse shows flutter waves. More often paroxysmal

Atrial fibrillation

- Most patients are asymptomatic but can complain of palpitation, dizziness or recurrent transient ischaemic attacks (cerebral microembolism).
- Associated rheumatic heart disease, dilated cardiomyopathy, MVP, ASD, IHD but often patient has a normal heart.
- Pulse is 160–250/min, irregularly irregular with pulse deficit (Table 5.6).
- ECG shows fibrillatory waves replacing P waves, though irregular QRS complexes are morphologically normal
- Emergent cardioversion is required if there is angina, haemodynamic compromise or hypotension.

- In haemodynamically stable patient treat by digoxin + propranolol or verapamil. Alternatives are quinidine and procainamide.
- When AF has high ventricular rate and wide QRS complexes – exclude WPW where digoxin, quinidine, verapamil are contraindicated; but procainamide/ disopyramide are preferable. Anticoagulation with aceumarol 2–4 mg daily/phenindiodone 50–150 mg daily/warfarin 2–10 mg daily to keep PT at INA of 2–3.

Table 5.7: Differentiation between VPB and AF

Features	Ventricular premature beats (VPBs)	Atrial fibrillation (AF)
Pulse deficit	Less than 10 per min.	More than 10 per min.
'a' wave in JVP	Present	Absent
On exertion	decreases or disappears	Persists or increases
Rhythm	Short pause (between normal beat and VPB) followed by a long pause (following VPB)	Pauses are variable and chaotic

6

NERVOUS SYSTEM

MIGRAINE

Essentials of diagnosis

- Lateralised episodic throbbing headache, often with photophobia, zig zags of light, scintillating scotomas, often positive family history.
- Basilar artery migraine—visual disturbances in both eyes, initially, accompanied or followed by dysarthria, disequilibrium, paresthesia, then occipital throbbing headache.
- Ophthalmoplegic migraine—transient external ophthalmoplegia with diplopia and headache.

Treatment

- Rest in a quiet dark room.
- Cafergot (ergotamine tartarate 1 mg + caffeine 100 mg) 1 tab every 30 minutes upto mxm 6 tab or rectal suppository 2 mg.
- Ergotamine 0.36 mg/puff; mxm 6 puffs in an attack or sublingual – mxm 6 mg or dihydroergotamine mesylate 1–2 mg SC/IM.
- Sumatriptan 6 mg SC or Zolmitriptan 2.5 mg PO.
- Propofol IV in intractable cases.
- Control of nausea with inj promethazine 50 mg or prochlorperazine 10 mg IV.
- Prophylaxis with drugs as for cluster headache (see below), inj. botulinum toxin to scalp.

CLUSTER HEADACHE

- Episodes of severe nocturnal unilateral periorbital pain, occurs daily for several weeks associated with nasal congestion, rhinorrhoea, lacrimation, redness of eyes and Horner's syndrome (transient).
- *Treatment* is with sumatriptan 6 mg SC or dihydroergotamine 1–2 mg or ergotamine tartarate aerosol or 100%, O_2, 7 L/min for 15 minutes; butorphanol 1 mg nasal spray to each nostril.
- *Prophylaxis* with ergotamine tartarate suppository 1 mg at night, propranolol 20–80 mg, methysergide 4–6 mg, verapamil 80–160 mg, clonidine 0.2–0.6 mg, armitryptyline 10–150 mg daily.

TRIGEMINAL NEURALGIA

- Sudden lancinating unilateral facial pain, triggered by touch, movement or eating along distribution of trigeminal nerve (second or third division).
- Can be idiopathic or symptoms of multiple sclerosis, brainstem neoplasm, CP angle tumor, aberrant vessel impinging on trigeminal nerve root.
- *Treatment* is with carbamazepine 600–1200 mg daily, dilantin 200–400 mg daily, gabapentin 900–1800 mg daily, often combined with baclofen 10–20 mg tid.
- If resistant to drugs–alcohol/glycerol injection to Gasserion ganglion, radio frequency rhizotomy, gamma radiosurgery to the trigeminal root, tractotomy and finally posterior fossa exploration for decompression.

EPILEPSY

Essentials of diagnosis

- Recurrent seizures–motor, sensory, autonomic, visual, auditory, gustatory, dysphasia, illusion, structured hallucinations, deja vu, jamais vu, affective disturbances; myoclonic jerks.

- Loss of consciousness, tongue bite, frothing, passage of urine and stool in grandmal seizure.
- Drop attack in atonic seizure, multiple myoclonic jerks; differentiate from pseudoseizure and vasovagal syncope (Table 6.1, 6.2).
- Postepileptic automatism, headache, sleepiness, often Todd's palsy.
- Typical EEG changes – spikes or sharp waves.

Treatment

a. Generalised tonic clonic and partial seizures — phenytoin 200–400 mg/d, carbamazepine 600–1200 mg/d, valproic acid 1500–2000 mg/d, phenobarb 100–200 mg/d, gabapentine/topirmate 200–400 mg/d, lamotrigine 100–500 mg/d, felbamate 1200–3600 mg/d, zonisamide 200–600 mg/d, tiagabine 2–56 mg/d.

Table 6.1: Differential diagnosis of hysterical fit (pseudoseizures) *vs* epileptic fit

Hysterical fit	Epileptic fit
Induced by emotional excitement.	Fairly constant periodicity.
Incontinence common.	No incontinece
Patient not hurt. Usually in presence of people.	Tongue biting. At times injury from fall.
Movements spectacular.	Can occur anywhere.
No clonic or tonic sequences	Tonic and clonic phases.
Plantar response down going.	Extensor plantar response.
Corneal reflex present.	Corneal reflexes absent during attack.
Pupils dilate.	Pupils remain unchanged.
No turning of head eyes, eyeballs roll upwards if eyes forcibly opened.	Conjugate deviation of and head and eyes.
Attacks may be prolonged to impress spectators.	Attacks of short duration
Recovery after attack sudden.	Gradual recovery.

Table 6.2: Seizure *vs* vaso vagal syncope

	Tonic-Clonic seizure	Vaso-Vagal syncope
Precipitant	Unusual	Emotional, painful or stressful event
Circumstances	Any	Usually upright posture, crowded or hot environment
Onset	Usually abrupt	Usually gradual with feeling of faintness, nausea, sweating, greying of vision
Motor phenomenon	Often character-istic tonic-clonic	Usually flaccid without movement
Skin colour	Pale or flushed	Pale
Breathing	Stertuous, foaming common	Shallow
Incontinence	Common	Unusual
Tongue biting	Unusual	Unusual
Vomiting	Common	Unusual
Injury	Drowsy, confused,	Common
Postictal	Headache, sleep	Rapid recovery
Duration of unconsciousness	Minutes	Seconds

b. Absence (petitmal) seizure — Ethosuximide 100–1500 mg/d, valproic acid, 1500–2000 mg/d, clonazepam 0.04–0.2 mg/kg.

c. Myoclonic seizure — valproic acid and clonazepam as above.

Felbamate causes aplastic anaemia and hepatic failure; hence blood count be done every 2–4 weeks. All newer epileptics are only adjuncts to established drugs except for lamotrigine.

TRANSIENT ISCHAEMIC ATTACK (TIA)

• Onset abrupt without warning and recovery occurs rapidly.

- Common symptoms of carotid TIA are weakness and heaviness of the arm, leg or face. Numbness and paresthesia may occur alone or in combination with motor deficit. Slowness of movement, dysphasia and monocular visual loss may occur.
- Examination may reveal carotid bruit, flaccid weakness-sensory changes, hyperreflexia, extensor plantar response.
- Vertebrobasilar TIA causes ataxia, vertigo, diplopia, dysarthria, dimness of vision, perioral numbness or paresthesia, weakness or sensory complaints on one, both, or alternating sides of the body.
- Carotid Doppler may show significant stenosis of internal carotid but CT is normal.
- *Treatment* is with IV heparin 5000–10000 IU followed by 1000–2000 IU/hr and introduction of warfarin 5–15 mg daily with discontinuation of heparin. Wafarin may be continued for a year. Alternatively aspirin 325 mg daily may be given from beginning. Those intolerant to aspirin be given ticlopidine 250 mg bid.
- Cigarette smoking be stopped; hypertension, hyperlipidemia, diabetes, arteritis, haematological disorders be treated appropriately. Aspirin/heparin prophylaxis in atrial fibrillation reduces chances of cerebral microembolism and TIA.
- In subclavian steal syndrome there is vertebrobasillar ischaemia with bruit in supraclavicular fossa, unequal radial pulse and a difference of above 20 mmHg between systolic BP in the arms.

STROKE

Essentials of diagnosis

- Sudden onset of characteristic neurologic deficit (see below).

- History of hypertension, diabetes, valvular heart disease, myocardial disease, atherosclerosis, increased thrombotic tendency, postpartum, etc.
- Lacunar syndrome include pure motor or sensory deficit, ipsilateral ataxia with crural paresis, dysarthria with clumsyhand syndrome; partial or complete recovery in 4–6 weeks is usual.
- Obstruction of carotid circulation causes amaurosis fugax (transient visual loss); anterior cerebral occlusion distal to its junction with anterior communicating artery causes weakness and cortical sensory loss in contralateral leg often with paratonic rigidity, grasp reflex, abulia (lack of initiative), urinary incontinence.
- *Middle cerebral trunk occlusion* leads to contralateral hemiplegia, hemisensory loss, and homonymous hemianopia. If dominant hemisphere is involved global aphasia occurs. Involvement of left anterior division causes expressive (Broca's) aphasia with contralateral palsy but only posterior division occlusion causes receptive (Wernicke's aphasia) and homonymous visual field defects. Involvement of non dominant hemisphere causes apraxia with contralateral palsy.
- *Posterior cerebral artery occlusion* causes thalamic syndrome, i.e. contralateral spontaneous pain and hyperpathia. Vertebral artery occlusion below the origin of anterior spinal and posterior inferior cerebellar is clinically silent unless other vertebral artery is congenitally small or atherosclerotic when syndrome similar to basilar occlusion occurs, unless circulation is compensated through circle of Willis. Posterior inferior cerebellar artery occlusion causes spinothalamic sensory loss involving face ipsilaterally, ninth and tenth cranial nerve palsy, limb ataxia and Horner's syndrome along with contralateral sensory loss.
- *Basilar artery occlusion* leads to coma, pinpoint pupils, flaccid quadriplegia and sensory loss and variable cranial nerve abnormalities. In hemiplegia of pontine

origin the eyes are deviated to paralysed side as opposed to deviation away from paralysed side in hemispheric lesion.

• Occlusion of major cerebellar arteries produces vertigo, . vomiting, nystagmus, ipsilateral limb ataxia and contralateral spinothalamic sensory loss. Massive cerebellar infarction may lead to tonsillar herniation, coma and death.

• CT scan is preferable to MRI in acute stage because intracranial haemorrhage is not easily detected in MRI within first 48 hours. However diffusion weighted MRI can detect ischaemia earlier than CT/standard MRI (Tables 6.3, 6.4).

Treatment

• When neurological deficit is progressive heparinization may limit infarct size provided CT is done to exclude expanding haematoma. tPA 1 mg/kg with 10% as bolus followed by 90% in 1 hour infusion is effective in reducing the neurologic deficit in patients without CT evidence of haemorrhage, provided given within 3 hours of onset of ischaemic stroke.

Table 6.3: MRI findings in cerebral infarction

Stage of infarction	MRI findings
Immediate	Intravascular contrast enhancement; Alteration of perfusion/diffusion coeficient
<12 hours	Anatomic changes of T1 images (gyral thickening,sulcal effacement, loss of grey-white interface)
12 to 24 hours	Hyperintensity, mass effect, Leptomeningeal enhancement
1 to 3 days	Obvious abnormality in T1 and T2 images (early parenchymal contrast enhancement, haemorrhagic transformation)

Table 6.4: CT findings in cerebral infarction

State of infarct	CT findings
Hyperacute (<1–2 hours)	Normal (50 to 60%), hyperdense artery (25 to 50%), obscuration of lentiform nuclei
Acute (12–24 hours)	Low density basal ganglia, loss of gray-white matter interface (insular Ribon sign), sulcal effacement
1–7 days	Mass effect, wedge shaped low density area involving white and grey matter, haemorrhagic transformation, gyral enhancement
1–8 weeks	Contrast enhancement persists, mass effect resolves
Months - years	Encephalomalacic change, volume loss, rarely calcification

- Brain edema (vasogenic) can be tackled with prednisolone upto 100 mg/dexamethasone 10 mg/day or dehydrating hyperosmolar agents.
- Blood pressure even if elevated be not reduced in acute phase as it may be reactive and may compromise circulation to ischaemic zone.
- Completed stroke only needs supportive therapy i.e. care of bladder, bowel, skin care, physiotherapy, joint mobility and nutrition along with long term aspirin or ticlopidine.
- Early mobilisation, speech rehabilitation and occupational therapy are essential. With severe and persisting motor deficit, leg brace and toe spring may help to increase mobility.

INTRACEREBRAL HAEMORRHAGE

Essentials of diagnosis

- Headache, vomiting gradually progressing to unconsciousness.

› Focal signs and symptoms depending upon site of bleed (see below). In thalamic haemorrhage there may be, in addition to motor deficit, loss of upward gaze, downward/skew deviation of the eyes, lateral gaze palsies and pupillary inequalities. In putaminal bleed besides motor deficit loss of lateral conjugate gaze is conspicuous. A hemisensory disturbance is also present with more deeply placed lesion. Cerebellar bleed has nausea, vomiting, headache, ataxia terminating in coma.

• CT scan (without contrast) determines site and size of haematoma.

Treatment

• Superficial haematoma in cerebral white matter causing mass effect and in cerebellar haematoma surgical evacuation is appropriate.
• Otherwise management is generally conservative and supportive.

Table 6.5: Differentiating various types of cerebrovascular disorders

Clinical	Embolism	Thrombosis	Haemorrhage
Features			
Age	Younger	Middle or old	Middle or old
Mode of onset	Acute	Insidious	Acute
Time of onset	Often during day	Often during sleep	Abruptly during day
History of			
1. Convulsion	Present	—	Present
2. Hypertension	—	—	Present
3. Cardiac lesion	Present	—	
Recovery pattern	Rapid recovery	Gradual	Delayed or no recovery
Prognosis	Good	Fair	Bad

Subarachnoid haemorrhage

- Sudden severe headache followed by vomiting and unconsciousness.
- Signs of meningeal irritation
- Focal deficit according to site of underlying lesion i.e. location
- CSF shows xanthochromia
- Hemiplegia or focal neurological deficit after 4–14 days due to focal arterial spasm.
- Subacute hydrocephalus after 2 weeks.
- Sentinel headache of warning leaks precede rupture of aneurysm
- In a-v malformation, besides haemorrhage symptoms may relate to cerebral ischaemia due to diversion of blood, or venous stagnation, distortion of adjacent brain tissue and gliosis, communicating and obstructive hydrocephalus.
- Seizure occurs in 20–40% of av malformation; tendency to bleed is more with smaller lesions.
- Cranial bruit is always an indication of a-v malformation
- *Treatment* of SAH is that of coma with respiratory, skin eye, bladder and bowel care; phenytoin prophylaxis against seizure; reduction of blood pressure gradually if elevated but diastolic not below 100 mmHg.
- Coil embolization/clipping is for aneurysm but excision is best for a-v malformation provided it causes rise in ICP, focal neurological deficit or bleeds. Inoperable av malformation needs gamma knife (induces sclerosis), placement of detachable balloons with their inflation with quickly solidifying contrast material or vasoocclusive polymer injection.
- Nimodipine 60 mg every 4 hour for 21 days may reduce vasospasm.
- Aminocaproic acid during first 14 days reduces the risk of recurrent haemorrhage but may increase the ischaemic complication.

• Any asymptomatic aneurysm more than 10 mm is to be treated surgically.

INTRACRANIAL TUMORS

Essentials of diagnosis

• Generalised and/or focal disturbances of cerebral function like personality changes, headache, seizure, focal deficits (see below).
• Increased intracranial pressure with herniation of temporal lobe uncus through tentorial hiatus compressing third cranial nerve, midbrain and posterior cerebral artery.
• Half of all primary intracranial neoplasms are gliomas and the remainder are meningiomas, pituitary adenoma, etc. Neurofibroma, haemangioblastoma and retinoblastoma have a familial tendency.
• The earliest sign is ipsilateral pupillary dilatation followed by decerebrate posturing and respiratory arrest. Herniation of cerebellar tonsils through foramen magnum causes medullary compression with apnea and circulatory collapse.
• *Frontal lobe lesions* — progressive intellectual decline, contralateral grasp reflex, focal motor seizure, contralateral pyramidal signs, anosmia, aphasia etc.
• *Temporal lobe lesions* — seizure with olfactory or gustatory hallucinations, lip smacking but without loss of consciousness, emotional and behavioral disturbances, déjà vu, jamais vu, micropsia, macropsia, auditory illusions and hallucinations. Left sided lesions may cause dysnomia and receptive aphasia and right sided lesions disturb musical notes and melodies.
• *Parietal lobe lesions* cause contralateral sensory disturbances like sensory seizure, inattention, sensory loss (cortical type with loss of vibration, posture and tactile discrimination). Lesions of left angular gyrus

cause Gerstmann's syndrome (alexia, agraphia, acalculia, finger agnosia, right-left confusion). Lesion of nondominant lobe cause dressing and constructional apraxia, anosognosia (denial, neglect or rejection of paralysed limb).

- *Occipital lobe lesions* cause crossed homonymous hemianopia, bilateral disease causes cortical blindness (loss of colour perception, prosopagonosia, i.e. inability to identify familiar face), simultagnosia (inability to interpret a composite scene), failure to turn eyes to a particular point in space, despite preservation of spontaneous and reflex eye movements – Balint's syndrome; and denial of blindness (Anton's syndrome).

- *Brainstem lesions* cause cranial nerve palsies, ataxia, incoordination, nystagmus, pyramidal and sensory deficit in limbs of one or both sides.

- *Cerebellar tumors* produce marked truncal ataxia with involvement of vermix; ipsilateral appendicular deficit (ataxia, incoordination, hypotonia) when cerebellar hemisphere are affected.

- CT scanning and gadolinium contrast enhanced MRI are diagnostic. MRI is preferred in posterior fossa and brainstem lesions. In plain CT meningioma is homogeneous and hyperdense located in parasagittal/sylvian region, olfactory groove, sphenoidal ridge, tuberculum sellae and enhances uniformly with contrast.

- *Treatment* depends upon site and type of tumor. In most cases treatment is surgical decompression followed by chemoradiotherapy. Ependymoma is radioresistant Brainstem gliomas are mostly inoperable.

- Shunting if tumor produces obstructive hydrocephalus
- Steroid support to reduce cerebral edema.
- Anti epileptic therapy to control seizure or as a prophylaxis against seizure either due to tumor or as a consequence of surgery.

- Primary cerebral lymphoma associated with HIV is indistinguishable from cerebral toxoplasmosis and is treated with whole brain radiotherapy.
- In single cerebral metastasis surgical removal may be possible in otherwise well patients.
- *Leptomeningeal metastasis* leads to multifocal neurological deficits with increased CSF pressure and protein, pleocytosis and decreased glucose; CT scan showing contrast enhancement in the basal cisterns or showing hydrocephalus without any evidence of mass lesion support the diagnosis. Treatment is irradiation to symptomatic areas combined with intrathecal methotrexate.
- *In spinal tumors* – pain is prominent with extradural lesions; characteristically aggravated by coughing and straining, often with sensory and motor deficits and sphincteric dysfunction. Intramedullary tumors (Table 6.6) are treated by decompression, surgical excision (when feasible) and by irradiation. Epidural spinal metastasis is treated with irradiation.

Table 6.6: Differentiation between intramedullary and exrtamedullary lesions of the cord

Features	Extramedullary	Intramedullary
Motor System		
1. Upper motor neuron sign	Common	Less common
2. Lower motor neuron signs		
i. Muscle atrophy	One or two segments at the site of root compression	Wide due to anterior horn involvement
ii. Trophic changes of the skin	Not common	Present
iii. Fasciculation	Rare	Common

Features	Extramedullary	Intramedullary
Sensory System		
1. Root pain	Common	Rare
2. *Funicular pain	Not present	Present
3. Dysesthesias and paresthesias	Rare	Common
4. Dissociated sensory loss	Absent	Present
5. Sacral sensation	Lost	Sacral sparing for pain and temperature
6. Joint position sense	Lost	Spared
7. Lhermitte's sign	Present	Absent
Autonomic Nervous System		
Bowel and bladder disturbances investigations	Late	Early
1. X-ray of the spine	Bony changes may be seen	Not seen
2. Effect of lumbar puncture	Signs and symptoms are precipitated or increased	Not such effect
3. Alteration in CSF	Frequently present	Absent
4. Manometry changes (Quecken Stedt's)	Early change	Late change

BRAIN ABSCESS

- Presents as an ICSOL, usually occurs secondary to rhinosinusitis, mastoiditis or systemic bacteremia.
- Headache, drowsiness, confusion, seizure are early symptoms followed by rise in intracranial pressure, and then focal neurological deficit.
- CT scan shows low density core with surrounding contrast enhancement, similar to tuberculoma and tumor.
- *Treatment* is with IV antibiotic combined with surgical drainage (aspiration or excision). Penicillin 2 mu IV 2

hrly plus metronidazole 750 mg IV 6 hrly plus chloramphenicol 1–2 gm IV 6 hrly is usually given for 6–8 weeks followed by orally for another 2–3 weeks; monitored with serial CT studies along with antiedema measures.

PSEUDOTUMOR CEREBRI

- Headache, diplopia.
- Papilledema, enlargement of blindspot, 6th nerve dysfunction.
- Normal CSF but under increased pressure.
- MRI venography may show sagittal or transverse sinus thrombosis.
- *Treatment* is with acetazolamide 250 mg tid with oral corticosteroids and repeated lumbar puncture to remove CSF. When medical treatment fails — subtemporal decompression, lumboperitoneal shunt or optic nerve sheath fenestration may be considered.

PARKINSONISM

Essentials of diagnosis

- Any combination of bradykinesia, rigidity, rest pill rolling tremor (Table 6.7) and postural instability; mild decline in intellectual function.
- Seborrhoea of scalp and face is common.
- Repetitive tapping over bridge of nose produces sustained blink response (Myerson's sign).
- Monotonous face with widened palpebral fissures, poorly modulated voice, micrographia, small suffling steps, unsteadiness on turning, difficulty in stopping and a tendency to fall.
- PET shows striatonigral hypometabolism.

Table 6.7: Parkinson's disease *vs* Huntington's chorea

	Parkinson's disease	Huntingtion's chroea
Site of neuronal loss	Pigmented nuclei	Caudate nucleus
Neurotrans-mitter loss	Dopamine	Acetylcholine (and GABA)
Excess of	Acetylcholine	Dopamine
Levodopa therapy	Improvement	Exacerbation of chorea
Phenothiazine	Exacerbation	Improvement

Treatment

- Anticholinergics – benztropine 1–6 mg daily, biperiden 2–12 mg daily, cycrimine 5–20 mg daily, procyclidine 7.5–30 mg daily, trihexyphenidyl 6–20 mg daily, orphenadrine 150–400 mg daily – reduce tremor and rigidity but not akinesia.
- Amantadine – 100 mg twice daily improves all features.
- Levodopa does not penetrate blood brain barrier and reduces peripheral breakdown of levodopa to dopamine. 4:1 ratio of levodopa: carbidopa is usually prescribed.
- COMT inhibitors – reduce metabolism of levodopa with more sustained plasma level of dopamine. Tolcapone 100–200 mg tid or entacapone is usually given. Serial liver function testing is mandatory with COMT inhibitors.
- Dopamine agonists — act directly on dopamine receptors — hence less chance of dyskinesia, on-off phenomenon. Bromocriptine 1.25 mg twice daily with gradual increase at 2 weeks interval to 10–30 mg daily and pergolide 0.05 mg daily with gradual built up are used in combination with low dose levodopa-carbidopa or alone. Pramipexole 0.125 mg tid and ropinirole 0.25 mg tid with gradual increase at weekly interval to optimal dose i.e. 0.5–1.5 mg tid and 2–8 tid respectively are also helpful.

- Selegiline, MAO-B inhibitors is adjunct to levodopa, given 5 mg at breakfast and 5 mg at lunch.
- Clozapine, an atypical antipsychotic without extrapyramidal effect, 6.25 mg at bed time increased to 25–100 mg/day reduces iatrogenic dyskinesia.
- Thalamotomy or palidotomy, on one side, when intolerant or unresponsive to medication.
- High frequency thalamic stimulation.
- Fetal adrenal medulla/substantia nigra transplantation into caudate nucleus may help.

MULTIPLE SCLEROSIS (MS)

Essentials of diagnosis

- Episodic neurologic symptom ranging from retrobulbar neuritis to numbness, tingling, weakness, spastic paraparesis, diplopia, sphincteric disturbance; relapsing and remitting course with incomplete recovery.
- Single pathologic lesion can not explain the clinical findings.
- Patient under 55 years of age at onset.
- MRI shows multiple foci of demyelination; evoked response studies may show subclinical involvement of visual, brainstem, auditory and somatosensory pathways.
- IgG oligoclonal band in CSF.

Treatment

- Prednisolone 60–80 mg daily for 1 week, then tappered over 2–3 weeks, preceded by methyl prednisolone 1gm IV for 3 days hasten recovery.
- For relapsing-remitting or secondary progressive disease beta interferon or glatiramere acetate SC daily reduce frequency of exacerbations.

- Immunosuppressants — azathioprine, cyclophospha- mide, methotrexate, mitoxantrone, cladribine arrest course of secondary progressive MS.
- Plasmapheresis, IVIg may help.
- *Treatment* of spasticity and bladder dysfunction if present.

MOTOR NEURONE DISEASE (MND)

Essentials of diagnosis

- Five types clinically — progressive bulbar palsy, pseudobulbar palsy, progressive spinal muscular atrophy (Table 6.8) primary lateral sclerosis, amyotrophic lateral sclerosis.
- In progressive spinal muscular atrophy degeneration of anterior horn cells of spinal cord produces LMN deficit but in primary lateral sclerosis there is purely UMN deficit while in amyotrophic lateral sclerosis there is mixed LMN and UMN deficit, often associated with dementia and parkinsonism.
- In progressive bulbar palsy there is drooping of soft palate, weak gas reflex, wasting and fasciculation of tongue. In pseudobulbar palsy (UMN lesion bilaterally) the tongue is spastic, contracted and can not be moved rapidly from side to side.
- In limbs – weakness, atrophy, fasciculation with increased reflexes but sensations are intact and sphincters are spared, CSF is normal
- EMG shows – abnormal spontaneous activity in resting muscles, reduction in number of motor units.

Treatment

- Riluzole which reduces presynaptic release of glutamate may slow progression of ALS.
- Symptomatic and supportive measures.

Table 6.8: Differentiation between SMA and motor neuron disease (progressive muscular atrophy)

Features	SMA	Progressive muscular atrophy
1. Family history	Present	Absent
2. Age of onset	2 to 20 years	Above 40 years
3. Pattern of involvement	Asymmetrical	Symmetrical
4. Bulbar muscle involvement	Not commonly	Usually involved
5. Deep tendon reflexes	Lost	Brisk
6. Progression	Slow	Rapid
7. Prognosis	Better	Worse

SYRINGOMYELIA

- Segmental atrophy and areflexia and loss of pain and temperature.
- Associated thoracic kyphoscoliosis.
- Pyramidal and sensory deficit in legs develop later and dysfunction of lower brainstem with bulbar palsy, nystagmus and sensory impairment over face may occur (syringobulbia).
- Associated Arnold-Chiari malformation (displacement of cerebellar tonsils, medulla and fourth ventricle), best seen in MRI, that also delineates extent of syrinx.
- *Treatment* is surgical decompression; suboccipital craniectomy and upper cervical laminectomy is done for Arnold-Chiari malformation; if cavitation associated with intramedullary tumor, radiation therapy may supplement surgery when complete removal is not possible.

BELL'S PALSY

- Lower motor neuron facial palsy (Table 6.9) of abrupt onset, angle of mouth is drawn to healthy side, ipsilateral eye closure is difficult, difficulty with eating and fine facial movements.

- Disturbance of taste in anterior 2/3rd due to involvement of chordatympani and occasionally hyperacusis due to palsy of stapedius.
- EMG, nerve excitability or conduction studies provide guide to prognosis.
- Prednisolone 60–80 mg/d for d 5 days followed by tapering the dose over next 10 days facilitates recovery if started within 5 days of palsy.
- Acyclovir therapy empirically since HSV of geniculate ganglion may be the pathology.
- Faradic stimulation, neostigmine may be helpful but decompression of facial canal is not of benefit.
- Protection of eye from exposure keratitis with patch.

Table 6.9: Facial palsy: UMN *vs* LMN

Upper motor neuron	Lower motor neuron
1. Affects mainly muscles of lower part of face, never complete.	Whole face affected, complete palsy.
2. Seldom isolated palsy.	Isolated paralysis.
3. Emotional movement preserved.	Loss of emotional movement.
4. No muscle contracture. contracture may occur.	Marked muscle
5. No reaction of degeneration	Reaction of degeneration present.
6. EMG and nerve conduction normal.	Evidence of lower motor neuron lesion in EMG.

MYASTHENIA GRAVIS

Essentials of diagnosis

- Fluctuating weakness of voluntary muscles producing ptosis, diplopia and difficulty in swallowing, chewing.
- Activity increases weakness of affected muscles.

- Short acting anticholinesterages (edrophonium) transiently improve the weakness.
- Often associated with thymoma, thyrotoxicosis, SLE, rheumatoid arthritis.
- Elevated level of acetyl choline receptor antibodies and decremental muscle response to stimulation in EMG; should be differentiated from Eaton Lambert myasthenia, secondary to bronchial carcinoma (Table 6.10).

Treatment

- Neostigmine 15 mg qid or pyridostigmine 60 mg qid
- Thymectomy if younger than 60 years, unless weakness is only restricted to extraocular muscles.
- Corticosteroids when above measures fail. Since weakness is initially aggravated by steroid – it be started in hospital stay and then switched on to alternate day therapy.

Table 6.10: The differences between myasthenia gravis and Eaton-Lambert syndrome

Features	Myasthenia gravis	Eaton-Lambert syndrome
1. Male: Female	3:2	1:1
2. Site of lesion	Postsynaptic	Presynaptic
3. Associated tumour	Thymic tumour	Oat cell carcinoma of the lung
4. Muscle power after exertion	Worsens	Muscle power may improve after first few contractions of muscle.
5. DTR	Preserved	Diminished or absent
6. Treatment with neo-stigmine or pyridos tigmine	Marked improvement	Slight improvement
7. Response to guanidine	No effect	Good response
8. Autonomic changes	No changes	Present

- Plasmapheresis and IVIg help in managing acute crisis and stabilising the patients before thymectomy.

BOTULISM

- The toxin prevents release of acetylcholine at neuromuscular junction and autonomic synapses causing muscle palsy. There is diplopia, ptosis, facial weakness, dysphagia, nasal speech. Pupils are dilated and unreactive. Paralytic ileus and postural hypotension.
- In EMG repetitive stimulation of motor nerves at fast rates increases muscle response.
- *Treatment* is with trivalent antitoxin 20,000 units; guanidine hydrochloride 25–50 mg/kg/d in divided doses may facilitate acetyl choline release from nerve endings.
- Respiratory assistance, may be necessary.
- Botulinum toxin is used in treatment of dystonia, blepharospasm, migraine, neuralgia, torticollis, anal fissure, entropion, facial cosmetic uplift and esophageal motility disorders, etc.

COMMON INFECTIOUS DISEASES

Common infectious diseases of the nervous system are listed in Table 6.11.

PURULENT MENINGITIS

- Fever, headache, vomiting, disturbed sensorium, neck and back stiffness, positive Kerning (Table 6.12) and Brudzinski signs.
- Low glucose, high protein, increased pressure and high polymorphs in CSF.
- Lumbar puncture be only performed if ICSOL is excluded by CT scan.

Table 6.11: Common infectious diseases of the nervous system

Type of infection	Time course of illness	Disease entity
Bacterial	Acute	Acute bacterial meningitis Recurrent meningitis Epidural abscess
	Chronic (eg Tubercular)	Chronic meningitis Brain abscess
Viral	Acute	Acute viral meningitis Acute viral encephalitis Post infectious encephalitis Acute transverse myelitis Cytome-galovirus Polyradiculitis
	Slow or chronic conventional agents	Retroviral: AIDS, HTLV-I/ TSP Progressive multifocal leukoence-phalopathy Subacute sclerosing panencephalitis (SSPE) Subacute measels encephalitis (SME) Progressive rubellaen-cephalitis (PRP) Entero viruses-Polio, Echo Others-CMV
	Prion diseases	Kuru Creutzfeldt-Jakob disease, etc.
Fungal Spirochetal Parasitic		Meningitis and abcess Neurosyphilis and Lyme disease. Protozoan-toxoplasmosis, cerebral malaria Helmenthic-neurocysti-cercosis, echinococcosis.

- Positive blood and CSF culture, organisms in CSF smear, latex agglutination diagnostic for encapsulated organisms – pneumococcus, meningococcus, *H. pneumonae* and cryptococcus).

- Pneumococci and meningococci respond best to cefotaxime 2 gm 6 hrly or ceftriaxone 2 gm bid IV. Alternatively penicillin G 3–4 MU every 4 hours IV can be given.
- When gram –ve bacilli or *L.monocytogenes* are suspected ampicillin 2 gm IV 4 hrly plus ceftazidime 50–100 mg/kg (upto 2 gm) every 8 hrly IV.
- Antiedema measures, prednisolone to retard meningeal adhesion
- Duration of therapy — *H. influenzae* and *N. meningitides* for 7 days, *S. pneumonae* for 10–14 days, *L. monoytogenes* for 14–21 days and gram negative bacilli for 21 days.

CHRONIC MENINGITIS

- Gradual development of symptoms over weeks to months.
- Most common pathogens — *M. tuberculosis*, Cryptococcus, meningovascular syphilis, *B. burgdorferi* (Lyme disease).
- In granulomatous meningitis (mycobacteria, fungi) CSF show lymphocytosis, with low glucose and high protein but in spirochetal meningitis CSF glucose is normal so also opening pressure.
- *Treatment* is tailored to infective agent.

Table 6.12: Differentiation between Babinski and pseudo Babinski sign

Babinski sign	Pseudo Babinski sign
1. Contraction of hamstring muscles can be felt	There is no associated contraction of the hamstring muscles
2. Pressure on the base of the great toe while eliciting the plantar reflex does not inhibit the extensor response	Pressure on the base of the great toe while eliciting the plantar response will inhibit the withdrawal extensor response

HERPES ENCEPHALITIS

- Flu-like syndrome followed by headache, fever, behavioral disturbance, seizure and coma.
- EEG — temporal lobe seizure foci.
- CT — temporal lobe mass effect, haemorrhagic lesion.
- HSV DNA PCR in CSF diagnostic.
- CSF — white cells and RBCs; brain biopsy diagnostic.
- *Treatment* is IV acyclovir 10 mg/kg 8 hrly for 10 days; valaciclovir and famciclovir are the alternatives.

ARBOVIRUS ENCEPHALITIDES

- Fever, sore throat, nausea, vomiting, convulsion, stupor, coma.
- Stiffness, meningeal irritation, tremors, convulsion, cranial nerve palsies, limb paralysis, absent superficial reflexes, exaggerated deep tendon reflexes, pathological reflexes.
- CSF glucose is normal, protein is increased, lymphocytic pleocytosis.
- Virus specific IgM or a four fold change in complement fixing or neutralizing antibodies.
- CT or MRI of brain showing basal ganglia or thalamic involvement or temporal lobe involvement – that exclude ICSOL or HSV encephalitis.
- *Treatment* is supportive and symptomatic. Reduction of raised ICT and monitoring of intraventricular pressure are essential. Antiviral therapy has no role.

LYMPHOCYTIC CHORIOMENINGITIS

- Influenza-like syndrome of fever, chills, cough followed by meningitis and stiffneck.
- Aseptic meningitis with positive Kernig's sign.
- CSF shows lymphocytic pleocytosis with slight increase in protein.
- *Treatment* is symptomatic and supportive.

Table 6.13: Virus encephalitis *vs* tuberculous meningitis

Characteristics	Virus encephalitis	Tuberculous meningitis
Fluid	Clear	Clear, may have fibrin web on standing
Pressure	Normal or increased	Normal or increased
Protein	Normal or increased	Increased. May be over 100 mg per cent
Glucose	Rarely below 40 mg. per cent. May be above 80 mg per cent, CSF/Blood ratio about 2/3	Usually in region of 20–25 mg. per cent. Rarely if ever above 45 mg. per cent CSF/Blood ratio < ½
Cells	May be normal. When increased usually of lymphocytes 50–200/cumm	
Organism	Some polymorphs in first week Bacteriologically sterile. Virus may be isolated.	Increased in first few weeks; polymorphs *Myco.tuberculosis* may be seen on microscopy. Direct culture may be positive in 6–10 weeks.
Antibodies	Antibody to particular virus may rise with serial samples	Gamma globulin increased.

ALZHEIMER'S DISEASE (AD)

- It is the most common degenerative dementia with progressive decline of cognitive function.
- Attention, memory, visuospatial processing, learning/ language are impaired.
- Depression, apathy, agitation and frank psychosis may occur.
- 5% cases are autosomal dominant with mutation of amyloid precursor protein (Chromosome 21) or presenilin protein I & II (Chromosome 14, 1).
- Amyloid plaques are an extra cellular accumulation of Ab and neurofibrillary tangles are intracellular paired helical structures containing tau protein. They are

present in hippocampus, amygdala, nucleus basalis, locus ceruleus, dorsal raphe nucleus.

- There is reduction in content of acetyl choline with reduced activity of choline acetyl transferase in fore brain.
- PET and SPECT imaging show bilateral hypoperfusion of posterior temporal and parietal lobes.
- CSF tau is increased, Ab is decreased.
- *Treatment* is with cholinesterase inhibitors – donepezil 5 mg – 10 mg daily; revastigmine 1.5 – 3 mg bid, galantamine 4–12 mg bid, huperzine 50–200 mg bid.
- Supportive therapy with Vit-E, Ginkgo biloba, selegiline (an MAO inhibitor); memantine (NMDA receptor antagonist) a chemical relative of amantadine, 40 mg per day modestly improves cognition.

Table 6.14: Differences between Alzheimer's disease and Pick's disease

Features	Alzheimer's disease	Pick's disease
Portion of brain	Diffuse cortical affected involvement (esp. hippocampus and temporal lobes)	Confined to frontal and temporal lobes (lobar sclerosis)
Pathology	Neurofibrillary tangles, Senile plaques seen	Pick's bodies seen
Age of onset	Presenile or senile	Presenile
Clinical Features	Features of diffuse cortical involvement seen; Fronto temporal features less prominent	Prominent fronto temporal features seen

GUILLAIN-BARRE SYNDROME (INFECTIVE POLY-NEURITIS)

- There are three major subtypes of GBS: (i) acute inflammatory demyelinating polyradiculoneuropathy,

(ii) acute motor-sensory axonal neuropathy and, (iii) acute motor axonal neuropathy.
- Miller–Fisher syndrome (ataxia, areflexia, ophthalmoplegia) is a variant of GBS.
- Recent infection with campylobacter, CMV, EBV, mycoplasma may antedate symptoms.
- Symptoms are mostly ascending – weakness, numbness, tingling in lower limbs, ascending up to trunk, arm and face.
- Weakness is symmetric affecting equally proximal and distal muscles.
- Pain and temperature are less affected than touch, vibration and position (large fiber).
- Tendon reflexes absent to decreased.
- Autonomic instability with hypo/hypertension, arrhythmia.
- Diagnosis is from motor and sensory conduction studies (delayed), absent to delayed F waves and H reflexes, raised CSF protein but normal cell count (albumino-cytological dissociation).
- *Treatment* is with IVIG 2 g/kg infused over 5 days or plasma exchange 250 ml/kg over 10–14 days.
- Respiratory failure occurs in 30% requiring ventilatory support.
- Disease progresses over 2–4 weeks and progression of symptoms and signs over 8 weeks excludes GBS.

Table 6.15: Differentiation between Guillain-Barré syndrome (GBS) and chronic inflammatory demyelinating polyneuropathy (CIDP)

Features	GBS	CIDP
Mode of onset Progression	Acute It evolves over days to weeks and then station-ary for several weeks	Insidious a. Slow and steady progression or stepwise manner b. Maximum severity after several months

7

DISEASES OF ALIMENTARY TRACT

UPPER GI BLEED

Essentials of diagnosis

- Haematemesis (bright red blood, or coffee ground).
- Melena in most cases, haematochezia if bleeding is massive.
- Postural hypotension and volume status determine severity of blood loss but haematocrit is a poor indicator in initial stages.
- Endoscopy is both diagnostic and therapeutic.
- Peptic ulcer disease, portal hypertension, Mallory-Weiss tear, erosive gastritis and vascular ectasia are the most common causes.

Treatment

- IV fluids (saline/Ringer lactate) or colloids; blood transfusion.
- Nasogastric aspiration and lavage with cold saline.
- In absence of continued bleeding haematocrit should rise 3% for each unit transfused packed red cells.
- IV ranitidine/omeprazole 80 mg/pantoprazole with 5% dextrose bolus, followed by infusion tid if erosive gastritis or peptic ulcer suspected.
- Desmopression 0.3 µg/kg IV in uremic bleed to improve platelet function.
- Octreotide 100 µg bolus followed by 50–100 µg/hr infusion for control of variccal bleed else sandostatin/

IV pitressin (contraindicated for CAD patients). If inescapable give with nitroglycerine.
- Injection of bleeding ulcer vessel with adrenaline, thermocoagulation or bleeding varices with sclerosing agents, tube compression of varices, their band ligation and even transvenous intrahepatic portosystemic shunts can be undertaken.
- Persistent bleeding from ulcer, angioma or Mallory-Weiss tears may demand intra arterial embolization or vasopression.
- Esophageal transection for uncontrollable varical bleed is rarely necessary.

Table 7.1: Differentiation between upper GI and lower GI bleed.

Features	Upper GI bleed	Lower GI bleed
Site	Above the ligament of Treitz	Below the ligament of Treitz
Presentation	Haematemesis/ malena	Haematemesis
Nasogastric aspiration	Blood	Clear fluid
BUN/Creatinine ratio	Increased (>25:1)	Normal (<25:1)
Bowel sounds	Hyperactive	Normal

LOWER GI BLEED

Essentials of diagnosis

- Haematochezia, in 10% cases it is due to upper GI bleed
- Evaluation with colonoscopy in stable patients when bleeding has stopped.
- Massive active bleeding calls for evaluation with sigmoidoscopy, upper GI endoscopy, angiography and nuclear bleeding scan (technetium labeled red blood scan).

- Spontaneous cessation of bleeding occurs in 85% cases and transfusion requirement is in < 40% cases.
- Infectious colitis, inflammatory bowel disease and anorectal disease account for younger patients; diverticulosis, vascular ectasia, malignancy or ischaemia in older patients.
- Painless large volume bleeding always suggests diverticulosis, bleeding from vascular ectasia; bloody diarrhoea associated with cramping, abdominal pain, urgency or tenesmus is characteristic of inflammatory bowel disease, infectious colitis or ischaemic colitis.

Treatment

- Stabilisation of patient with crystalloid and blood transfusion.
- Therapeutic colonoscopy – injection or cautery of bleeding lesions or high risk lesions.
- Intra arterial embolization of ectasia or intraarterial vasopression, both helpful in diverticular bleed or bleeding vascular ectasia.
- Surgery is indicated in patients with continued bleeding requiring more than 4–6 units of blood in 24 hours or more than 10 units. Most such haemorrhages are due to vascular ectasia or diverticular disease demanding resection of bleeding segment of intestine or colon. When accurate localization is not possible or when emergency surgery is required for massive haemorrhage total abdominal colectomy with ileorectal anastomosis is required.

GASTROESOPHAGEAL REFLUX DISEASE

Essentials of diagnosis

- Heart burn, often exacerbated by meals, bending or recumbency.

- Atypical manifestations like asthma, chronic cough, chronic laryngitis, sore throat, noncardiac chest pain, periodontitis and enamel erosion.
- Odynophagia and dysphagia when there is peptic stricture.
- Endoscopy shows erythema and friability of lower esophageal mucosa and erosions; but barium swallow is not helpful.
- Ambulatory esophageal pH monitoring and GE sphincter manometry are diagnostic.

Treatment

- Avoid lying down within 3 hours of meal; 6" elevation of head end of bed.
- Avoid acidic foods – tomato products, citrus fruits, coffee, spicy food and agents that relax LES, delay gastric emptying (fatty food, alcohol, chocolate, smoking); small frequent meals.
- Antacids – H_2 receptor blockers or proton pump inhibitors for 8–12 weeks, e.g. ranitidine 150 mg, famotidine 20 mg, nizatidine 150 mg twice daily or omeprazole 20 mg, lansoprazole 30 mg, pantoprazole 40 mg or rabeprazole 20 mg once daily.
- Promotility drugs – Cisapride, mosapride, etopride, metoclopramide and bethanecol that enhance esophageal peristalsis increase LE sphincter tone and improve gastric emptying.
- Proton pump inhibitors, however, remain the drug of choice for severe erosive disease and H_2 – antagonists for mild disease. Patients with severe erosive esophagitis, Barrett's esophagus or peptic stricture should be maintained on longterm proton pump inhibitors. Dose can be doubled if once daily dose is insufficient to suppress acid secretion.
- Patients who are unresponsive require laparoscopic fundoplication.

- Endoscopy therapy (1) endoscopic "sewing machine" to place sutures below GE junction creating mucosal plication, (2) endoscopic radiofrequency therapy, (3) submucosal glue injection.

INFECTIOUS ESOPHAGITIS

- Common to immunosuppressed patients.
- Symptoms of odynophagia, dysphagia and chest pain.
- Endoscopy with biopsy establishes the diagnosis. Endoscopic findings in candidal esophagitis are diffuse, linear yellow white plaques adherent to mucosa. In CMV esophagitis there are large superficial ulcerations. Oral lesion may be present in patients of HSV esophagitis.
- *Treatment* of candidal esophagitis is with nystatin 500,000 units swallow 5 times daily for 7–14 days or fluconazole 100–200 mg orally daily. Nonresponders need low dose amphotericin B 0.3–0.5 mg/kg/day. Initial therapy of CMV esophagitis is with ganciclovir 5mg/kg IV bid for 3–6 weeks and that of herpetic esophagitis is with acyclovir 250 mg/m^2 IV bid/tid for 7–10 days.

CAUSTIC ESOPHAGEAL INJURY

- Severe burning, chest pain, gagging, dysphagia and drooling after ingestion of caustic/acid, accidental/ suicidal.
- Aspiration results in stridor and wheezing.
- Maintain circulation by IV fluid and airway patency.
- Endoscopy be done within 24 hours to assess mucosal damage. If damage is mild liquid diet by nasoenteral tube.
- Patients with severe injury i.e. deep or circumferential ulcers or necrosis run the risk of perforation, bleeding and stricture. They need IV alimentation for 2 days followed by nasoenteral feeding and then liquid diet as per tolerability.

- Esophageal stricture if develops needs repeated dilatation.
- Patients of severe esophageal injury if deteriorate warrant emergency surgery with esophagectomy and colonic/jejunal interposition.
- Antibiotics and steroids are not required.
- Esophageal malignancy remains a danger demanding surveillance.

ESOPHAGEAL VARICES

- One third of patients with varices develop upper GI bleed.
- Varices are found in 50% of patients with cirrhosis, secondary to portal hypertension.
- Varices per se do not cause dyspepsia, dysphagia or retching.
- Diagnosis is established by upper GI endoscopy and barium swallow.
- *Treatment* of varices is (1) band ligation, (2) sclerotherapy, (3) portosystemic shunt surgery, (4) transvenous intrahepatic portosystemic shunt, (5) betablockers and long acting nitrates.

CANCER ESOPHAGUS

- Progressive dysphagia for solid foods over weeks to months.
- Odynophagia is sometimes present.
- Significant weight loss.
- Local tumor extension causing tracheoesophageal fistula, recurrent nerve palsy, mediastinitis etc.
- Endoscopy with biopsy establishes the diagnosis.
- Stage III ($T_3N_1M_0$ or T_4 any N & M) and stage IV (any N or T with M_1) disease need palliation by palliative resection, radiotherapy, stent placement, photodynamic therapy and endoscopic laser therapy (NdYAG).

- Stage IIA disease needs esophagectomy but very small tumors may be treated by endoscopic mucosal resection, alternatively patient can be offered with radiotherapy plus chemotherapy (5 FU + Cisplatin).
- In stage IIB and IIIA surgical resection be followed by chemoradiotherapy.

ACHALASIA

- Gradual progressive dysphagia for solids and liquids.
- Regurgitation of undigested food, nocturnal regurgitation causes cough and aspiration.
- "Bird beak" distal esophagus in barium swallow; smooth, symmetric.
- Esophageal manometry confirms the diagnosis i.e. complete absence of peristalsis, incomplete LES opening with swallowing.
- Substernal chest pain in half the cases and weight loss.
- *Treatment* is by (1) endoscopy guided botulinum toxin injection, (2) pneumatic dilatation, (3) modified Heller's cardiomyotomy (laparoscopic).

ESOPHAGEAL DYSMOTILITY

- Dysphagia and chest pain; dysphagia is intermittent and nonprogressive. Dysphagia often provoked by stress, large bolus of food, hot or cold liquids.
- Chest pain may mimic angina but is non exertional.
- Cork screw esophagus in barium swallow.
- Esophageal manometry may show diffuse esophageal spasm, nut cracker esophagus, hypertensive lower esophageal sphincter, etc.
- *Treatment* is with oral nitrates or nitroglycerine sublingually; calcium channel blockers; botulinum toxin injection; Maloney bougies dilatation; and lastly long surgical myotomy.

GASTRITIS AND GASTROPATHY

- Consists of erosive and haemorrhagic gastritis, nonerosive nonspecific gastritis and specific types of gastritis with distinctive endoscopic and histologic features. Erosive gastritis causes epigastric pain, nausea, anorexia and vomiting and often haematemesis; best diagnosed by endoscopy.
- Stress gastritis, NSAID gastritis, alcoholic gastritis, portal gastropathy all belong to erosive gastritis
- *H. pylori* gastritis, gastritis of pernicious anaemia and lymphocytic gastritis are non erosive-non specific gastritis. *H. pylori* is best diagnosed by ELISA for antibody, fecal antigen immunoassay, ^{14}C urea breath test or endoscopic biopsy.
- Proton pump inhibitors be discontinued 14 days prior to *H. pylori* tests. *H. pylori* predisposes to gastric malignancy, MALT lymphoma and initiates and maintains peptic ulcer disease.
- Pernicious anaemia gastritis severely affects fundal glands with their atrophy, intestinal metaplasia. Parietal cell antibodies directed against $H^+K^+ATPase$ pump are invariable.
- Chronic granulomatous inflammation (TB, syphilis, sarcoid, Crohn's disease, fungal), bacterial (phlegmonous or necrotising gastritis), viral (CMV) eosinophilic, lymphocytic and hypertrophic (Menetrier disease) gastritis are not uncommon.
- Hypertrophic gastropathy is characterised by giant thick gastric folds involving body causing nausea, epigastric pain, weight loss, chronic protein loss often requiring gastric resection.
- Erosive and stress gastritis is treated by H_2 receptor blockers and proton pump inhibitors. If bleeding occurs, their continuous infusion and sucralfate suspension orally are indicated (1 gm every 4–6 hours).
- *H. pylori* is treated with any of the following regimes for 10–14 days.

1. Proton pump inhibitor twice daily + clarithromycin 500 mg twice daily + metronidazole 500 mg twice daily.
2. Bismuth citrate 400 mg twice daily + Clarithromycin 500 mg twice daily + metronidazole 500 mg twice daily/ tetracycline 500 mg twice daily.
3. Proton pump inhibitor twice daily + bismuth subsalicylate 2 tablets 4 times daily + tetracycline 500 mg 4 times daily + Metronidazole 250 mg 4 times daily.

- NSAID induced gastritis can be reduced by prophylactic use of proton pump inhibitor or misoprostol 200 µg 3–4 times daily.

Table 7.2: Differentiating chronic gastritis from peptic ulcer

Chronic gastritis	Peptic ulcer
History of repeated attacks of acute gastritis	History of ingestion of NSAIDs
Pain slight, more soreness Pain intensified by food, No pain if meal is delayed.	Pain usually severe. Food may relieve pain
Pain relatively constant Symptoms of indigestion marked Slight or no haemorrhage Endoscopy: Patchy mucosal irregularity	Intermissions Few symptoms of indigestion Profuse hematemesis Endoscopy: Ulcer with creamy base

PEPTIC ULCER DISEASE

Essentials of diagnosis

- Non-specific epigastric pain with variable relationship to meal.
- Ulcer symptoms characterised by periodicity and rhythmicity; particularly in duodenal ulcer.
- 10–20% of patients present with ulcer complications (haemorrhage, perforation, obstruction, malignancy) without antecedent symptoms.

- Endoscopy is most diagnostic, antral biopsy for *H. pylori* is essential.
- Gastric ulcer biopsy or documentation of complete healing is necessary to exclude gastric malignancy.
- Alcohol and dietary factor usually do not cause ulcer disease; role of stress is also uncertain.
- Pain is aggravated by meal in gastric ulcer and food relieves pain in duodenal ulcer. Vomiting is common in gastric ulcer but a late feature in duodenal ulcer caused by gastric outlet obstruction.
- Nocturnal pain is more common in duodenal ulcer.
- Serum gastrin estimation is essential to exclude Zollinger Ellison syndrome (gastrinoma); testing for *H. pylori* is mandatory.

Treatment

- Proton pump inhibitors – rabeprazole 20 mg, esmeprazole 20 mg, pantoprazole 40 mg, lansoprazole 30 mg, 30 minutes before breakfast daily for 4 weeks in duodenal ulcer and 8 weeks in gastric ulcer.
- H_2 receptor antagonists — less effective and need longer duration of therapy, e.g. ranitidine 150 mg bid, roxatidine 150 mg bid, famotidine 20 mg bid, nizatidine 150 mg bid.
- Sucral fate — 1 gm 4 times daily. Bismuth subsalicylate — 2 tab three times daily.
- *H. pylori* eradication reduces ulcer recurrence.
- Refractory ulcers need exclusion of gastrinoma, gastric malignancy masquerading as ulcer.
- Surgery is indicated for persistent refractory ulcers.

Complications of Peptic Ulcer

1. ***Bleeding*** — see upper GI bleed.

2. ***Ulcer perforation***

   Develops in 5% of ulcer patients; usually silent causing bacterial peritonitis, sepsis and shock.

Patient appear ill with rigid quiet abdomen, rebound tenderness, upright film shows gas below diaphragm.
- *Treatment* is laparoscopic perforation closure with omental patch, lavage of peritoneal cavity proximal vagotomy and treatment of of *H. pylori* to reduce recurrence.

3. Ulcer penetration

- Change in intensity and rhythmicity of ulcer symptoms, i.e. pain becomes more severe and constant, may radiate to back and is unresponsive to drugs. Such patients be tried with IV H_2 blockers/proton pump inhibitors and if do not improve laparotomy be performed.

4. Gastric outlet obstruction

- Occurs due to edema or cicatricial narrowing of the pylorus or duodenal bulb.
- Symptoms are early satiety, heaviness after meals followed by projectile vomiting, the foul smelling vomitus containing food ingested even day before, ending in severe malnutrition, metabolic alkalosis.
- *Treatment* is IV saline and KCl to correct metabolic acidosis; nasogastric decompression of stomach.
- Endoscopy be done to exclude neoplasm, and to do hydrostatic balloon dilatation.
- Unresponsive patients be offered surgery — vagotomy with pyloroplasty or antrectomy.

ZOLLINGER-ELLISON SYNDROME

- Peptic ulcer disease, multiple ulcers and severe symptoms, ulcers at atypical sites (Jejunum, Meckel's diverticulum).
- Gastric acid hypersecretion (BAO>15 mEq/hr).
- Hypergastrinemia > 1000 pg/ml; when level less — secretin stimulation test be done.
- Diarrhoea very common, relieved by nasogastric suction.

- Somatostatin receptor cintigraphy and endoscopic US more dependable than CT, MRI; 80% gastrinomas occur in gastrinoma triangle bounded by porta hepatis, neck of pancreas and third part of duodenum. Localised disease needs resection even if lymphnode metastasis is present. In presence of hepatic metastasis, acid hypersecretion be controlled with proton pump inhibitors in higher dose followed by expectant treatment since the tumor is slow growing.

CARCINOMA STOMACH

- Dyspeptic symptoms with weight loss in patients above 40 years.
- Iron deficiency anaemia, occult blood in stool.
- Upper GI endoscopy diagnostic but CT and endoscopic US be done to know depth of invasion and nodal/distant spread.
- Can present with haematemesis (ulcerative lesion) or gastric outlet obstruction or dysphagia due to lower pyloric/lower esophageal obstruction.
- *Treatment* is with curative resection for stage I-III disease but those with hepatic or distant metastasis be offered palliation with single agent (5 FU) or combination chemotherapy (5 FU, cisplatin, doxorubicin). Palliative resection of the tumor removes risk of bleeding and obstruction. In unresectable tumor, gastrojejunostomy may be needed to prevent obstruction. Bleeding or obstruction from unresected tumors may be treated with endoscopic laser, or stent, radiation or angiographic embolisation.

GASTRIC LYMPHOMA

- Presentation is with dyspepsia, weight loss or bleeding
- Endoscopy shows an ulcer, mass or diffusely infiltrating lesion. Endoscopic biopsy shows proliferation of CD19

and CD20 positive lymphocytes (mucosa associated lymphoid tissue) differentiating primary nodal lymphoma infiltrating stomach wall.

- All MALT lymphoma be tested for *H. pylori* and if positive anti *H. pylori* therapy be instituted. Patients of stage IE (localised to stomach wall) or II E (adjacent lymph node involved) who are *H. pylori* negative or fail to respond to anti *H. pylori* therapy be offered surgical resection or local irradiation or both. Those with distant metastasis or high grade lymphoma be given CHOP regime chemotherapy.

MALABSORPTION

- Clinically manifest with steatorrhea (bulky light coloured stool), diarrhoea, weight loss, abdominal distention, vitamin deficiency (megaloblastic anaemia), iron deficiency anaemia, paresthesia, tetany (vit D, calcium deficiency), bleeding tendency (vit K deficiency), edema (protein loss), etc.

- In celiac sprue there is greasy stool with increased fecal fat, abnormal small bowel biopsy (loss of villi), positive antigliadin/anti endomysial antibodies and improvement on gluten free diet (wheat, rice, barley eliminated) and avoidance of dairy products (associated lactose intolerance).

- In Whipple's disease there is fever, arthralgia, lymphadenopathy, multisystem involvement (myocarditis, valvular regurgitation, uveitis, retinitis, seizure); duodenal biopsy shows PAS positive macrophages containing gram positive *T. whippelii*. Treatment is with TMP-SMX, one DS tablet daily for 1 year. Those unresponsive may respond to interferon gamma.

- In bacterial overgrowth (following achlohydria, diabetic pseudo obstruction, chronic pancreatitis), prior GI surgery symptoms of malabsorption are evident and jejunal aspirate has organisms above 10^5/ml and ^{14}C-xylose breath test is positive. Treatment is with ciprofloxacin 500 mg twice daily, norfloxacin 400 mg bid or TMP-SMX DS twice daily plus metronidazole 400 mg bid.

- In lactose deficiency patients have bloating, abdominal cramp and flatulence with milk and milk products. Hydrogen breath test is positive. Treatment is with lactose restriction and lactase supplement.

PARALYTIC ILEUS

- Abdominal discomfort with nausea, vomiting, obstipation, constipation.
- Minimal abdominal tenderness, decreased to absent bowel sounds.
- Precipitating factors include – surgery, peritonitis, electrolyte abnormalities (K^+, Ca^{++}, Mg^{++}), severe medical illness (pneumonia, uremia, ketoacidosis), drugs (anticholinergics, opioids).
- Air fluid levels and distended gas filled loops of small and large intestine in plain x-ray abdomen.
- *Treatment* is nasogastric suction, maintenance of nutrition, correction of electrolyte abnormality and treatment of precipitating event of peritonitis (perforation, pancreatitis, strangulation), infection and sepsis and electrolyte abnormality. Peritonitis secondary to peritoneal spillage needs higher broad spectrum antibiotics, peritoneal lavage. Colonic perforation runs the risk of growing anaerobes and clostridia in fertile peritoneal sac.

APPENDICITIS

- Early periumbilical pain, later right lower quadrant pain and tenderness, anorexia, obstipation, often vomiting.
- Low grade fever and leukocytosis, guarding in right lower quadrant with rebound tenderness.

- The psoas sign (pain on passive extension of right hip) and obturator sign (pain on passive flexion and internal rotation of right hip) are strongly suggestive.
- Microscopic haematuria and pyuria may be present in one fourth cases.
- Abdominal and transvaginal US is helpful and CT scan is useful to exclude periappendiceal abscess following perforation.
- Atypical presentations — urgency of defecation and urination in pelvic appendicitis; minimal abdominal signs in retrocecal appendicitis, subtle symptom is aged and very young.
- *Treatment* of uncomplicated appendicitis is surgical (laparoscopic). If perforation or abscess occurs antibiotics (amoxycillin + clavulanate or third generation cephalosporin along with metronidazole) followed by surgery after 6 weeks is recommended. Abscess can be drained under CT guidance.

INTESTINAL TUBERCULOSIS

- Mucosal ulceration with scarring leading to obstruction; mostly at ileocecal region causing weight loss, diarrhoea, chronic pain abdomen; ileocecal mass may be palpable.
- Complications include intestinal obstruction, haemorrhage, fistula formation and bacterial overgrowth with malabsorption.
- Barium radiography may show mucosal ulceration, thickening or stricture formation. The ileocecal region is drawn up due to thickening of mesentery.
- *Treatment* is with standard antituberculous regime.

IRRITABLE BOWEL SYNDROME (IBS)

- Chronic functional disorder characterised by abdominal pain, relieved by defecation, alteration in bowel habits, more frequent stools, loose stools.

- Lower abdominal pain is crampy, intermittent, worse 1–2 hours after meals; mucous with stool is usual.
- Weight loss, haematochezia, fever, nocturnal diarrhoea negate diagnosis of IBS.
- *Treatment* is with dietary modification, i.e. avoidance of flatulogenic foods like bean, cabbage, sprouts, cauliflower, raw onion, coffee, red wine and beer; high fiber diet.
- Drug treatment includes – antispasmodics (dicyclomine 10–20 mg tid; hyosciamine 0.125 mg orally/SL), antidiarrhoeals–lopereamide 2 mg tid; diphenoxylate with atropine 2.5 mg tid; GI motility stimulants in spastic type IBS like metochlopramide/cisapride 10 mg tid; antidepressants-desipramine 25 mg bed time, setraline 50–150 mg or fluoxetine 20–40 mg daily.

ANTIBIOTIC ASSOCIATED COLITIS

- Symptoms vary from mild to fulminant disease, attributable to *C. difficile.*
- Stool toxin assay for diagnosis is most dependable.
- Flexible sigmoidoscopy shows pseudomembrane only in severe cases; nonspecific colitis in mild-moderate cases.
- Abdominal pain, fever, leukocytosis, mucus and little blood in stool but profuse watery diarrhoea in severe cases. Fecal leukocytes are present only in 50% cases.
- X-ray may show mucosal edema and thumbprinting.
- *Treatment* is with metronidazole 500 mg tid for 10–14 days or vancomycin 125 mg qid raised to 500 mg qid. In severe cases IV metronidazole be given but IV vancomycin does not penetrate the bowel.

CROHN'S DISEASE

Essentials of diagnosis

- Intermittent low grade fever, non-bloody diarrhoea, right lower quadrant pain, mass and tenderness.

- Perianal disease with abscess, fistula.
- Narrowing of small intestine due to inflammation, spasm and fibrosis causing obstructive symptoms.
- Increased incidence of cholelithiasis due to malabsorption of bile salts and nephrolithiasis.
- Extraintestinal manifestations like — episcleritis, oligo articular non deforming arthritis, erythema nodosum, pyoderma gangrenosum, sclerosing cholangitis and cholangio carcinoma.
- Anaemia due to chronic inflammation, mucosal blood loss, iron deficiency, and vitamin B_{12} malabsorption; hypoalbuminemia due to intestinal protein loss.
- Colonoscopy shows segmental involvement with linear or stellate ulcers, biopsy shows granulomatous lesions.
- PANCA is usually negative but ASCA (antibodies to yeast *S. cerevisiae*) positive.

Treatment

- Maintenance of nutrition with adequate vitamins, proteins, low fat, medium chain triglyceride supplemented with low roughage diet.
- Control of diarrhoea with cholestyramine 2–4 gm or colestipol 5 gm 2–3 times daily before meals. Loperamide and tincture of opium may be used.
- Sulfasalazine 1.5–2 gm twice daily is effective in colonic involvement and mesalamine in small bowel involvement.
- Corticosteroid – 1 mg/kg for 2–3 weeks, then 5 mg reduction in dose/week followed by maintenance of 5–10 mg daily. An abscess be ruled out by CT before starting steroids.
- Ciprofloxacin 500 mg bid (better for ileitis) or metronidazole 10 mg/kg/day (better for colitis).

- Azathioprine 2–2.5 mg/kg and mercaptopurine 1–1.5 mg/kg when unresponsive to steroid.
- Infliximab (IgG anti TNF antibody) 5 mg/kg IV, best suited to bring rapid improvement while azathioprine effect takes place.
- Intractable disease, obstruction, massive bleeding may require surgical intervention, i.e. resection.

Table 7.3: Distinguishing Features Between intestinal Tuberculosis and Crohn's Disease

Features	Tuberculosis	Crohn's disease
Clinical		
1. Duration	Months	Years
2. Course	Continuous	Remission and Exacerbations
3. Fever	Common	Less common
4. Diarrhoea	Common (consti -pation may occur)	Very common
5. Lump abdomen	Palpable	Not palpable
6. Ascites	Common	Uncommon
7. Fistulae (internal and external)	Rare	Common
8. Rectal and peri-rectal fistula	Rare	Common
9. Pulmonary lesion	May be present	Not present
10. Anal lesions	Rare	Common
11. Miliary nodes on serosa	Common	Rare
12. Length of stricture	Small	Long
13. Ulcers	Annular	Serpiginous
14. Caseation	Usually Present	Absent
15. Acid fast bacilli	Often present	Absent
16. Fibrosis	Common	Very common

ULCERATIVE COLITIS

Essentials of diagnosis

- Bloody diarrhoea – mild < 4/d, moderate 4–6/d, severe · > 6/d.
- Lower abdominal cramp, fecal urgency, tenesmus.
- Anaemia, low serum albumin.
- Negative stool culture.
- Periods of symptomatic flare ups and remissions.
- Sigmoidoscopy/colonoscopy shows mucosal edema, friability, mucopus and erosions.
- Extracolonic manifestation – erythema nodosum, pyoderma gangrenosum, episcleritis, thromboembolism, oligoarticular nondeforming arthritis, sclerosing cholangitis, cholangiocarcinoma.

Treatment

- Proctitis – mesalamine suppository 500 mg twice daily + hydrocortisone suppository 100 mg daily.
- Proctosigmoiditis – mesalamine enema 4 gm daily + hydrocortisone enema 100 mg daily.
- Mild to moderate extensive colitis – Sulfasalazine 1.5–3 gm PO twice daily or mesalazine 2.4–4 gm/d or olsalazine 0.75–1.5 gm PO twice daily. If no response after 4 weeks add prednisolone 40–60 mg/d, taper 5 mg/ week.
- Severe extensive colitis – Methyl prednisolone 48–60 mg IV daily or hydrocortisone 300 mg in 4 divided doses PO/by infusion or ACTH 120 units/d. IV cyclosporin to those not responding to steroid. If no response in 10 days – surgery (total proctocolectomy)
- Fulminant colitis and toxic megacolon – (colonic dilation of > 6 cm, toxemia, hypovolemia, bleeding) give broad spectrum antibiotic, nasogastric suction, IV fluids and treat as for severe extensive colitis.
- If no improvement in 72 hours or there is worsening – surgery be performed before perforation.

Table 7.4: Differentiation of ulcerative colitis from Crohn's disease

	Ulcerative colitis	Crohn's disease
History		
Smoking	Non smokers	Smokers (more severe)
Family history	Occasionally	15–20%
Clinical		
Bloody diarrhoea	Common	Not so common
Abdominal lump	Rare	Common
Perianal disease	Uncommon	Frequent
Signs of malabsorption	Never	Frequent
Radiology		
Distribution	Continuous	Segmental
Mucosa	Fine ulceration	'Cobblestones'
Colonoscopy/ Sigmoidoscopy	Double contour Loss of vascular pattern, contact bleeding, ulceration and spontaneous bleeding	'Rose-thorn' ulcers Deep longitudinal ulcers, skip lesions
Histology		
Distribution	Mucosal	Transmural
Cellular infiltrate	Polymorphs, plasma cells, eosinophils	Lymphocytes, Macrophages
Glands	Destroyed	Preserved
Complications	Toxic dilatation, carcinoma	Stricture, abscess, fistula, malnutrition, B_{12} deficiency, short bowel syndrome, gallstones, renal stones

DIVERTICULOSIS/DIVERTICULITIS

- Abdominal pain, and fever.
- Left lower abdominal tenderness and mass.
- Positive stool occult blood, leukocytosis.
- Micro perforation (most common) with paracolic inflammation or macroperforation with either abscess or generalised peritonitis may occur.

- May result in stricture of colon, bleeding and fistula formation to bladder, bowel and vagina.
- Sigmoidoscopy and barium enema are diagnostic but are not to be done in acute stage for fear of perforation.
- *Treatment* of mild acute diverticulitis is with low residue diet, metronidazole 500 mg tid plus ciprofloxacin 500 mg bid for 14 days. Moderate to severe disease is managed by IV fluids, nil orally and metronidazole/ clindamycin plus aminoglycoside else piperacillin-tazobactam/ticarcilin clavulanate can be used.
- Large abscess, peritonitis need emergency surgery but those with fistulas or colonic obstruction require elective surgery. The diseased segment can be resected and reanastomosed.

COLONIC POLYPOSIS

- Can be adenomatous (most common) and hyperplastic (of no clinical consequence).
- Non familial adenomatous polyps can be tubular, villous or tubulovillous, the villious form having high malignancy potential.
- Small polyps cause positive occult blood and large polyps haematochezia; diagnosis is by barium enema/ sigmoidoscopy or colonoscopy.
- *Treatment* is by colonoscopic polypectomy, followed by periodic colonoscopic surveillance.
- Familial adenomatous polyposis is due to APC gene mutation and colorectal cancer is inevitable by 50 years unless prophylactic colectomy is done.
- Hamartomatous polyposis syndromes include (1) Peutz Jeghers syndrome (small intestinal polyps, pigmented buccal mucosa) - causing bleeding, intussusception, obstruction, (2) familial juvenile polyposis (high malignancy potential), (3) Cowden's syndrome (extensive polyposis but innocuous).

COLORECTAL CANCER

- Symptoms and signs dependent upon tumor location (1) proximal colon – anaemia, fecal occult blood; (2) distal colon – change in bowel habit, bleeding per rectum.
- Rectal cancers – tenesmus, urgency, recurrent bleed.
- Barium enema, colonoscopy diagnostic.
- Resection is the treatment of choice, with regional lymphnode dissection. Adjuvant therapy with pelvic radiation and 5FU for stage II and stage III disease. Metastatic disease needs palliation with 5FU, leucovorin and irinotecan.

HAEMORRHOIDS

- Bright red blood per anum, perineal discomfort but inflammation, thrombosis or infarction cause acute severe pain.
- Mucoid discharge in chronically prolapsed haemorrhoids.
- *Treatment* is with high fiber diet; band ligation or sclerotherapy for stage I and II; excision for stage III or IV disease. Medical treatment consists of quinolones to control infection, analgesics, calcium dobsilate, diosomine, etc.

8

HEPATOBILIARY DISEASES

VIRAL HEPATITIS

Essentials of diagnosis

- Prodrome of anorexia, nausea, vomiting, malaise, flu syndrome.
- Fever, enlarged tender liver, jaundice (Table 8.1).
- Leukopenia, abnormal liver function tests (raised aminotransferases).
- HBV infection often is associated with arthritis, glomerulonephritis and polyarteritis nodosa.
- IgM antibodies to hepatitis A are diagnostic, HBsAg disappears with appearance of anti HbsAg. HbeAg indicates viral replication and infectivity and its persistence in serum beyond 3 months indicates chronic hepatitis B.
- HCV is diagnosed from presence of anti HCV which is not a protective antibody.
- HGV, also transmitted percutaneously like HBV, HCV and HDV; causes chronic viremia lasting at least 10 years without significant liver disease.

Treatment

- Bed rest; palatable meals without much fat.
- 10% glucose if vomiting is pronounced.
- Gradual return to activity in convalescene.
- Phytotherapy as liver protectives, *L*-ornithine have no defined role.
- In cholestatic phase of acute hepatitis A, steroid wash out may be effective.

- In acute hepatitis C-interferon alfa enhances recovery and prevents progression to chronic hepatitis.
- Prophylaxis is with vaccine 1 ml IM with booster at 6 months for hepatitis A and with 3 doses of 20 µg each at 0,1,6 months for hepatitis B. Over 80% of all patients with acute hepatitis C progress to chronic hepatitis and ultimately 30% of them develop cirrhosis. 40% of those with chronic hepatitis B develop cirrhosis; and those with persistent HbeAg are at increased risk of hepatocellular carcinoma. Immunoglobulin 0.02 ml/kg is protective against HAV contacts and HBIG 0.06 ml/kg for HBV contacts.

Table 8.1: Differentiation of various forms of jaundice

Features	Hemolytic	Hepatocellular	Obstructive
1. Mechanism	Increased bilirubin production	Hepatocellular failure	Bile duct obstruction
2. Common cause	Hemolysis	Virus, drugs	Ca pancreas, gall stones
3. Mode of onset	Rapid	Gradual	Gradual
4. Symptoms	Anaemia, fever	Anorexia, nausea, vomiting Distaste to cigarette, coffee	Recurrent abdominal colic Fluctuating jaundice
5. Skin tinge	Mild yellow tinge	Orange	Greenish yellow
6. Urine (absent bile pigments)	Colourless	High coloured	Dark coloured (Presence of bile pigments)
7. Urobilinogen	++	+	Absent
8. Pruritus	Nil	+	+++
9. Bradycardia	Nil	Rare	+
10. Motion	Normal	Pale	Clay coloured
11. Serum bilirubin	Unconjugated	Both Conjugated & Unconjugated)	Conjugated

(Table 8.1 contd.)

Features	Hemolytic	Hepatocellular	Obstructive
12. AST & ALT	Normal	Grossly elevated	Slightly elevated
13. Serum alkaline phosphatase	Normal	Slightly raised	Grossly elevated
14. Coomb's test	Positive	—	—
Osmotic fragility	Increased	—	—
15. Spleen	++	+/-	-
16. Gall bladder	Not palpable	Not palpable	Palpable

ACUTE HEPATIC FAILURE

- Half the cases are due to HBV; 1–2% of acute HBV progress to chronic HBV and acute hepatic failure in less than 1%.
- Fulminant hepatic failure is occurrence of hepatic encephalopathy within 8 weeks of onset of hepatitis. Coagulopathy is invariable. Hepatitis C is a rare cause of acute hepatic failure.
- Besides hepatitis acute liver failure can occur due to Reye's syndrome, fatty liver of pregnancy, shock, hepatic malignancy (usually lymphomas), drug reaction, mushroom poisoning, etc.
- Jaundice may be absent or minimal but aminotransferase are markedly raised except for Reye syndrome (microvesicular steatosis) where enzyme rise is modest.

Treatment

- Aimed at managing coagulation defect, fluid and electrolyte disorder, renal failure, hypoglycemia, sepsis and control of encephalopathy.
- Prophylactic antibiotic to reduce secondary sepsis.

- Acetyl cystine 140 mg/kg followed by 70 mg/kg PO 4 hrly, not only for paracetamol poisoning but for FHF of any cause.
- Mannitol 100–200 ml (20%) over 10 minutes to reduce brain edema provided there is no renal failure.
- Lactulose orally 30 ml thrice daily or 300 ml retention enema, to convert gut ammonia to nonabsorbable ammonium salt.
- Suppression of NH_3 producing gut flora with neomycin 0.5 gm 6 hrly or vancomycin 1 gm twice daily.
- Restriction of dietary protein to < 10 gm/day.
- When agitation is marked oxazepam 10 mg (not metabolised by liver)
- Sodium benzoate 10 gm/d and ornithine asparate 9 gm tid may help to reduce ammonia.
- Benzodiazepine competitive antagonist flumazenil IV may help.
- Zinc deficiency, if present, be corrected.
- Associated renal failure (hepatorenal syndrome) may respond to infusion of ornipressin and albumin, dopamine, octreotide and midodrine.
- Hepatic assist devices – extracorporeal whole liver perfusion
- Emergency hepatic transplant – in stage II/III encephalopathy.

CHRONIC ACTIVE HEPATITIS

- Chronic persistent hepatic inflammation beyond 3–6 months with raised aminotransferases and characteristic histologic findings (piece meal necrosis, periportal inflammatory cell infiltration).
- Can be graded to minimal, mild, moderate and severe; besides viruses can be autoimmune (positive ANA, smooth muscle antibody, anti LKM1 with raised IgG), drugs (INH, methyl dopa), alfa$_1$ antitrypsin deficiency.
- *Treatment* of HBV CAH is with interferon alfa 2b, 5 million units daily/10 million units altday IM for 4

months; alternatively with lamivudine 100 mg daily PO for 1 year with viral clearance in each case of 40%.

- HDV CAH may respond to IFN alfa 2a 9 MU thrice a week for one year.
- HCV CAH responds best to pegylated 1FN 180 mg once a week for 48 weeks or alfa 2a/2b 3MU three times a week for 24 weeks along with ribavirin 1000–1200 mg/d in two divided doses. Non-responders to interferon may do well with interleukin – 1O.

ALCOHOLIC HEPATITIS

- Symptoms range from asymptomatic patient with enlarged liver to acute liver failure with ascites, tender hepatomegaly, splenomegaly, jaundice, fever and encephalopathy.
- Leukocytosis, macrocytic anaemia less often thrombocytopenia (direct toxic effect of alcohol or hypersplenism); raised AST more than ALT, raised alkaline phosphatase and GGTP, raised serum bilirubin, and prolonged bleeding time, low serum albumin and raised globulin, increased hepatic iron store.
- Liver biopsy shows macrovesicular fat, PMN infiltration with hepatic necrosis, Malloy bodies and micronodular cirrhosis.
- *Treatment* is with abstinence from alcohol with nutritional support (protein, vitamins and calories); methyl prednisolone 32 mg/d for one month, Pentoxiphylline 400 mg orally tid for 1 month.
- Oxandrolone, (S) adenosyl-l-methionine, propylthiouracil are experimental.

HEPATIC STEATOSIS (FATTY LIVER)

- Besides alcohol, amiodarone, corticosteroids, methotrexate cause macrovesicular steatosis so also obesity, NIDDM.

- Tetracycline, valproic acid, anti HIV drugs cause microvesicular steatosis
- Impaired responsiveness of fat cells to insulin, increased leptin, and TNF α in obesity contribute to nonalcoholic fatty liver disease (NAFLD).
- US shows hyperechoic liver parenchyma; ALT rise is more than AST.
- *Treatment* of NAFLD is weight loss if obese, fat restriction, ursodeoxycholic acid 15 mg/kg/day; insulin sensitizers (pio/rosiglitazone), vitamin E and phlebotomy (to reduce oxidative stress.
- Cirrhosis only occurs in upto 5% of cases).

CIRRHOSIS OF LIVER

Essentials of diagnosis

- Weight loss, fatigue, weakness, muscle cramp, anorexia, abdominal pain (stretching of Glisson's capsule), loss of libido, impotency, gynaecomastia.
- Enlarged firm liver with a blunt or nodular edge, the left lobe may predominate.
- Skin manifestations – spider naevi (in upper body), palmar erythema, mild jaundice may be there; parotid enlargement, Dupuytren's contracture.
- Hypoalbuminemia with ascites, peripheral edema, pleural effusion occur late.
- Hepatic encephalopathy occurs late with day-night reversal, asterixis (liver flap), drowsiness, tremor (often precipitated by GI bleeding, high protein diet, diuresis, sepsis).
- Signs of portal hypertension, i.e. splenomegaly, ascites, esophageal and rectal varices, dilated veins on abdomen and thorax, caput medusae.
- Often fever due to cholangitis, spontaneous bacterial peritonitis.
- Laboratory features of hepatic decompensation; CT, Doppler US document hepatic nodules, ascites, patency

of portal, hepatic and splenic veins; endoscopy documents varices and biopsy is diagnostic – fibrosis, regenerating nodules.

Table 8.2: Features of postnecrotic *vs* alcoholic cirrhosis

	Postnecrotic	Alcoholic cirrhosis
Sex	More common in females	More common in males
Age	Any age	Usually middle age
Previous hepatitis	Frequent	Rare
Liver	Small or normal	Large
Spleen	Usually palpable	Not palpable in about 75%
Ascites	+ +	+
Heamatemesis (oesophageal varices)	Frequent	Uncommon
Hepatic coma	Common	Rare
Pyrexia	Rare	Common
Obesity	Rare	Common
Special features	Nil	Delirium tremens, Peripheral neuritis, Parotid enlargement Dupuytren's contracture. Wasting of muscle mass.

Treatment

- High carbohydrate high protein diet with vitamins.
- Management of ascites and edema with diuretics (spironolactone 100 mg daily but monitor for hyperkalemia); large volume paracentesis, peritoneovenous shunts, TIPS, etc.
- SBP (ascitic fluid > 500 cells/cmm) is treated with cefotaxime 2 gm tid IV or ceftriaxone.
- See hepatic encephalopathy for treatment.
- Anaemia and haemorrhagic tendency is treated with iron, folic acid and vitamin K supplement/fresh frozen plasma.

- Hepatopulmonary syndrome (increased A-a gradient, Rt to Lt intrapulmonary shunt due to a-v communication within lung) causes dyspnoea in upright position; treated by methylene blue that inhibits nitric oxide induced vasodilation, reversed also by liver transplantation.
- Liver transplantation.

BILIARY CIRRHOSIS

- Insidious onset, jaundice, raised alkaline phosphatase, (Table 8.3) pruritus.
- Steatorrhoea, xanthoma, xanthelasma, osteomalacia, osteoporosis, portal hypertension.
- Association of other autoimmune diseases like – Sjogren syndrome, dysthyroidism, scleroderma, celiac disease.
- Positive antimitochondrial antibodies; biopsy shows – portal inflammation with granuloma, bile duct proliferation, fibrosis.
- *Treatment* is with cholestyramine 4 gm or colestipol 5 gm three times daily: rifampin 150 mg bid, naltrexone 50 µ/day PO, UDCA – 10–15 mg/kg/day, colchicine 0.6 mg twice daily, methotrexate 15 mg PO weekly – all intended to retard hepatic fibrosis.
- Calcium, vitamin A,D,K, calcium supplementation; estrogen and bisphosphonates for osteoporosis; ondansteron may be helpful in improving general well being.

PRIMARY SCLEROSING CHOLANGITIS

- Progressive obstructive jaundice with pruritus, steatorrhoea, anorexia, raised alkaline phosphatase.
- Positive ANCA, some may have HIV, positive anticardiolipin antibodies and positive rheumatoid factor.

Table 8.3 : Features of postnecrotic cirrhosis *vs* biliary cirrhosis

	Postnecrotic cirrhosis	*Biliary cirrhosis*
Incidence	Common	Rare
Age	40–60	Any
Sex	Male	Female
Malnutrition	Frequent	Rare
Jaundice	Uncommon, mild	Always present, marked
Liver	May be small	Always markedly enlarged
Spleen	Enlarged	Slight enlargement
Ascites	Frequent	Rare and late
Xanthomas	Absent	May be seen
Alkaline phosphatase	Not raised	Raised
Serum cholesterol	Normal or diminished	Elevated
Mitochondrial antibodies	Absent	Antimitochondrial antibody (AMA) present
Autoimmune disorders	Nil	Present (RA, diabetes, thyroid disturbances, Sjogren's syndrome)

- ERCP and MRCP diagnostic, distinguishing ductopenia with cholestasis but normal cholangiogram.
- *Treatment* is with UDCA, balloon dilatation or stent placement for localised stricture, surgical excision of stricture and liver transplantation.

HEPATOCELLULAR CARCINOMA

- Associated with cirrhosis in general, HCV, HBV in particular. Think of it when deterioration occurs in otherwise stable cirrhotic; there is sudden bloody ascites (portal-hepatic vein thrombosis by tumor).

**Table 8.4: Laboratory findings in obstructive
vs parenchymal liver disease**

Test	Obstructive liver disease	Parenchymal liver disease
1. AST and ALT	Mild increase	Moderate to marked increase
2. Alkaline phosphatase	Markedly increased	May be mildly increased
3. Serum albumin	Normal	Decreased
4. Prothrombin time	Normal	Increased
5. Bilirubin	Normal or increased	Normal or increased
6. GGT	Increased	Normal or increased
7. 5' nucleotidase	Increased	Normal

- Cachexia, weightloss, weakness; tender enlarged liver often with a bruit and friction rub.
- Leukopenia as opposed to leucocytosis of cirrhotic patient.
- Raised haematocrit in one third due to ↑ eythropoitin
- Raised alfafetoprotein, MRI/helical CT diagnostic.
- *Treatment* is resection or liver transplantation but chemoembolisation, radiofrequency ablation can be under taken.
- Risk of hepatocellular carcinoma in cirrhotic is 3–5 % per year.

CHOLELITHIASIS

- Often asymptomatic, discovered in US, 15% stone are radiopaque, can present with biliary colic (right upper quadrant pain), cholangitis or intestinal obstruction (gallstone ileus). *Treatment* is laparoscopic chole-cystectomy. Chenodeoxy cholic acid and UDCA are bile salts when given for 2 years in doses of 7–13 mg/kg day in 3 divided doses may dissolve floating small gall stones in a functioning gall bladder. Lithotripsy in combination with bile salt therapy for single radiolucent gall stone less than 2 cm in diameter is often employed.

- Cholesterolosis is usually asymptomatic and needs no treatment. Adenomyomatosis may cause biliary colic and when symptomatic demands cholecystectomy.

CHOLECYSTITIS

- Steady severe pain and tenderness in right hypochondrium often radiating to right infrascapular region or pain in epigastrium with fever, nausea, vomiting.
- Positive Murphy's sign, leukocytosis.
- Palpable gall bladder and jaundice in some; latter often due to impacted cystic duct stone (Mirizzi's syndrome).
- Mild aminotransferase rise, often due to cholangitis.
- HIDA scan shows impacted cystic duct stone but abdominal US is not specific.
- Severe inflammation can lead to gangrene of GB (muscle guarding) or cholangitis (Charcot's triad of fever with chill, right upper quadrant pain and jaundice).
- *Treatment* is nil orally, IV fluids and alimentation, analgesics (meperidine preferred over morphine for fear of spasm of sphincter of Oddi) and antibiotics against *E. coli*. Once inflammation subsides laparoscopic cholecystectomy be performed. In high risk patients US guided aspiration of GB may postpone surgery.
- Following cholecystectomy, dilatation of cystic dust remnant, *foreign body granuloma*, neuroma formation in ductal wall, or traction on CBD by a long cystic duct remnant can cause persistent pain. Removal of cystic duct remnant may be necessary.
- Biliary dyskinesia due to elevated pressure in sphincter of Oddi as demonstrated in biliary manometry may cause pain mimicking cholecystitis. Endoscopic sphincterotomy, botulinum toxin injection into the

sphincter, calcium channel blockers and long acting nitrates bring relief.

CHOLEDOCHOLITHIASIS

- Can present as painless progressively increasing jaundice.
- Sudden severe right upper quadrant pain radiating to right shoulder and scapula.
- History of or concurrent features of cholangitis — fever with chills, jaundice, gram negative shock, hypothermia, leukocytosis
- US shows dilated CBD; MRCP shows the stone.
- CBD stone lasting longer than 30 days causes liver dysfunction progressing to cirrhosis; hence endoscopic papillotomy with stone extraction be done.
- Choledocholithiasis discovered during laparoscopic cholecystectomy may need removal of stone laparoscopically.
- In choledocholithiasis complicated by ascending cholangitis urgent ERCP, sphincterotomy and stone extraction be done with control of cholangitis with ciprofloxacin 250 mg IV bid /gentamicin 1.5 mg/kg tid.
- When choledochostomy is done for stone removal, T tube decompression of CBD is necessary and the tube be removed after 3 weeks after performing T tube cholangiogram.

ACUTE PANCREATITIS

Essentials of diagnosis

- Acute deep epigastric pain, radiating to back; better in sitting and leaning forward, made worse by walking and lying supine.
- Nausea, vomiting, sweating and weakness.
- Fever, abdominal distention and tenderness, mild jaundice.

- Tachycardia, hypotension, cold-clammy skin often present.
- History of alcohol intake, heavy meal or biliary stone disease.
- Leukocytosis, proteinuria, granular casts, hyperglycemia, elevated serum amylase and lipase, abnormal coagulation tests, decrease in serum calcium.
- Ascites and left pleural effusion may complicate and have high amylase content.
- Rise in C-reactive proteins, palpable upper abdominal mass indicate pancreatic necrosis.
- Paralytic ileus with diminished to absent bowel sounds.
- Contrast CT most dependable for knowing extent of necrosis; presence of gas bubbles indicate infection by gas forming organisms; CT guided aspiration confirms infection.
- Complications include volume depletion, ileus, renal failure, ARDS, pancreatic abscess, pseudocyst, pancreatic ascites, intra abdominal haemorrhage due to vessel erosion.

Treatment

- Nil orally, IV fluids, maintenance of blood pressure.
- Meperidine 100–150 mg IM 3–4 hrs to control pain.
- Fresh frozen plasma for coagulopathy.
- IV calcium gluconate if there is hypocalcemia with tetany.
- Antibiotics – Cefuroxime 1.5 gm IV tid, then 250 mg PO bid or Imipenem 500 mg IV tid.
- Necrotising pancreatitis needs surgical debridement.
- Chronic pseudocyst requires endoscopic/ percutaneous catheter or surgical drainage.
- Multiorgan failure may occur in severe haemorrhagic pancreatitis demanding proper vigilance and lexipafent, an antagonist of platelet activating factor.

CHRONIC PANCREATITIS

- Persistent or recurrent episodes of epigastric and left upper quadrant pain with referral to upper left lumbar region.
- Anorexia, nausea, vomiting, flatulence, constipation, weight loss.
- Tenderness over pancreas, mild muscle guarding and paralytic ileus during recurrences.
- Steatorrhoea (bulky foul fatty stools).
- Normal amylase does not exclude the diagnosis; but amylase and lipase are usually increased during acute attacks.
- Plain x-ray shows pancreatic calcification, CT scan shows calcification as well as ductal dilatation and atrophy of pancreas, but ERCP/MRCP more dependable.
- *Treatment* is with low fat diet, abstinence from alcohol, pancreatic enzyme supplement, H_2 receptor blockers/ proton pump inhibitors to decrease lipase inactivation, treatment of associated diabetes, octreotide 200 µg SC thrice daily often relieves pain.
- Surgical – total/subtotal pancreatectomy to reduce pain, repair of strictured pancreatic duct, removal of stone.

9
DISEASES OF BLOOD

IRON DEFICIENCY ANAEMIA

- Features of anaemia like palpitation, breathlessness, tachycardia.
- Skin and mucosal changes – koilonychia, smooth tongue, brittle nail, cheilosis.
- Dysphagia due to esophageal web (Plummer Vinson syndrome).
- Microcytic – hypochromic blood picture with increased iron binding capacity, decreased serum iron, absent stainable iron in marrow, increased transferin receptors
- In severe deficiency – raised platelets, target cells, pencil-shaped cells.
- *Treatment* is with oral iron – ferrous sulphate 325 mg tid providing 180 mg of elemental iron of which 18 mg is absorbed and therapy be continued for 3-6 months to replenish tissue stores after attaining normal haemoglobin.

Parenteral iron is for those not tolerating oral iron or there is urgency. Iron-dextran or iron sorbitol is given deep IM or the total calculated dose is given as infusion over 4-6 hours (1 gm storage iron +1 mg for each ml decrease in RBC mass below normal).

THALASSEMIAS

- Microcytosis out of proportion to the degree of anaemia
- Abnormal redcell morphology with target cells, acanthocytes.
- Positive family history.
- Raised HbA_2 and often HbF in betathalassemia.

- *In betathalassemia major* – no HbA is present and major Hb is HbF with basophilic stippling with nucleated red blood cells in peripheral smear.
- Betathalassemia minor resembles iron deficiency except for basophilic stippling and raised HbA_2.
- Expansion of marrow to compensate ineffective erythropoiesis with wide medullary cavity, bossing and sun-ray appearance of skull, hepatosplenomegaly, osteopenia, bony deformity and pathologic fractures.
- *Treatment* is with folate supplement, regular transfusion, stem cell/bone marrow transplantation; SC desferoxamine or oral kelfer to chelate excess of transfused iron, hydroxyurea for promoting HbF synthesis.

MEGALOBLASTIC ANAEMIA

- Macrocytic anaemia with megaloblastosis in marrow.
- Hypersegmented neutrophils in peripheral smear.
- Low serum B_{12} (< 100 pg/ml) and low folate.
- Neuropsychiatric changes, peripheral neuropathy, degeneration of posterior cord in B_{12} deficiency.
- Raised LDH, increased bilirubin, hyperplastic bone marrow.
- Intestinal malabsorption.
- Decreased intrinsic factor and gastric mucosal atrophy in pernicious anaemia with increased intrinsic factor antibodies and propensity for gastric malignancy.
- *Treatment* is vitamin B_{12} 100 μg IM daily for first week, weekly for first month and then monthly. Oral cobalamin dose is 1000 μg daily. Large dose of folic acid may improve anaemia of vitamin B_{12} deficiency but will worsen neurologic symptoms.

SPHEROCYTOSIS

- Positive family history, splenomegaly.
- Spherocytes and increased reticulocytes, decreased haptoglobin.

- Pigmented gall stones with attacks of cholecystitis.
- Aplastic crisis due to folate lack or infection.
- Microcytic hyperchromic indices.
- Splenectomy is the treatment with regular folate supplement.
- Paroxysmal nocturnal haemoglobinuria.
- Episodic haemoglobinuria causing reddish brown urine particularly in morning since respiratory acidosis of sleep enhances complement activity and haemolysis.
- Increased vulnerability to mesenteric and hepatic vein thrombosis.
- As it is a stem cell disorder it can progress to aplastic anaemia, myelodysplasia or AML.
- Low leukocyte alkaline phosphatase, absence of CD_{59} in flowcytometry.
- *Treatment* is with iron supplement; alternate day prednisolone or else bone marrow transplantation if there is transformation to myelodysplasia.

SICKLE CELL ANAEMIA

- Sickled cells in peripheral smear.
- Chronic haemolytic anaemia — mild icterus, reticulocytosis, decreased haptoglobin, pigment gall stones.
- Acute painful vaso-occlusive episodes causing back pain, leg pain, priapism, minor stroke brought about by dehydration, infection, hypoxia.
- Renal papillary necrosis with haematuria, shrunken spleen due to repeated infarction.
- Increased susceptibility to infections, nonhealing leg ulcers, hepatomegaly, retinopathy.
- Increased level of HbF, and higher its level – more benign is the course.
- *Treatment* is folic acid supplement, maintenance of hydration, exchange transfusion for vaso-occlusive crisis, hydroxyurea 500 mg daily to increase HbF,

pneumococcal vaccination (for hyposplenism) and bone marrow transplantation.

AUTOIMMUNE HAEMOLYTIC ANAEMIA

- Spherocytes and reticulocytosis in peripheral smear.
- Positive Coomb's test for IG autoantibody.
- Anaemia of rapid onset with fatigue, often angina and CHF.
- Jaundice and splenomegaly are usual.
- *Treatment* is with prednisolone 1-2 mg/kg/day; if ineffective splenectomy be done. When both ineffective immunosuppression with cyclophosphamide, azathioprine, or cyclosporin.
- High dose IV Ig 1 gm daily best controls haemolysis, though short term.

APLASTIC ANAEMIA

- Pancytopenia (reduced red cells, platelets and leukocytes).
- No abnormal cells in peripheral smear.
- Hypocellular bone marrow leads to neutropenia, frequent bacterial infections, and thrombocytopenia leads to mucosal and skin bleeding.
- Hepatosplenomegaly, lymphadenopathy and bone tenderness are always absent.
- Supportive treatment is antibiotic prophylaxis and component transfusion. Younger patients be treated with bone marrow transplantation but those above 50 years be given immunosuppression with ATG 6 mg/kg/d for 4 days combined with prednisolone 1mg/kg and cyclosporine 4 mg/kg twice daily can lead to transfusion free life.
- Oxymetholone 2-3 mg/kg daily.
- Cyclophosphamide 200 mg/kg/day has low response rate.

POLYCYTHEMIA VERA

- Increased red blood cell mass (PCV > 60%, Hb > 18 gm%).
- Increased platelets and leukocytes usually.
- Splenomegaly, normal arterial oxygen saturation.
- Increased blood viscosity causes headache, dizziness, tinnitus, blurred vision, fatigue; epistaxis, pruritus after warm shower (histamine release).
- Increased transcobalamine III and vitamin B_{12} activity.
- *Treatment* is phlebotomy (500 ml) weekly to reduce PCV to below 45%, myelosuppression with hydroxyurea 500-1500 mg daily; allopurinol for hyperuricemia; aspirin and anagrelide as antiplatelet and radioactive phosphorus (now rarely used).

MYELOFIBROSIS

- Leukoerythroblastic blood picture, giant abnormal platelets.
- Tear drop poikilocytes on peripheral smear.
- Striking splenomegaly; anaemia, bone pain, bleeding; hepatomegaly in half due to extramedullary erythropoiesis causing portal hypertension, ascites .
- Increased reticulin in fibrotic marrow.
- *Treatment* is with oxymetholone 200 mg daily; splenectomy, component transfusion, alpha interferon 2-5 mu SC three times a week; bone marrow transplantation.

CHRONIC MYELOID LEUKEMIA (CML)

Essentials of diagnosis

- Strikingly elevated white blood cell count (1.5 lac/cmm), predominant metamyelocytes with a low percentage of promyelocytes and blasts in peripheral smear.
- Positive philadelphia chromosome or *bcr-abl* gene.
- Hypermetabolic state with fever, nightsweat, fatigue
- Splenomegaly causing abdominal fullness; sternal tenderness.

- Hypercellular marrow with blasts < 5%.
- Low leukocyte alkaline phosphatage score, ↑ trans-cobalamine III.
- In blast phase – myeloblasts exceed 30% in marrow.
- Extreme leukocytosis can cause priapism, visual blurring, respiratory distress, confusion.

Treatment

- Emergent leukapheresis with myelosuppressive therapy when count is very high.
- Hydroxyurea 500-2500 mg/day or imitanib mesylate (tyrosine kinase inhibitor).
- Alpha interferon 5 mu/m^2/day SC for 5 years.
- Bone marrow transplantation in young.

Table 9.1: Differences between myelodysplastic syndromes and myeloproliferative disorders

Features	Myelodysplastic disorders	Myeloproliferative disorders
Splenomegaly	Absent	Present
Blood counts	Usually low	Usually high
Basophilia	Absent	Present
Marrow:		
Cellularity	Increased	Markedly increased
Dysplasia	Present	Mild or absent
Fibrosis	Absent	May be present
Cytogenetics	-7, +8, 5q and others	t(9:22) in CML, sporadic non-diagnostic abnormalities in other disorders.
Transformation rate to AML	High if marrow blasts > 5%	High in CML, low in other disorders.
Treatment	Increases counts: by transfusions and hemopoietic growth factors	Reduce counts by phlebotomy/ leucopheresis, platelet pheresis, cytotoxic agents.

MYELODYSPLASIA

- Peripheral cytopenia with hypercellular marrow
- Morphologic abnormalities in two or more haematopoietic cell lines.
- Hypogranular platelets, neutrophils have usually bilobed nucleus with scant granules.
- Dwarf megakaryocytes with unilobed nucleus in marrow
- Anaemia treated by transfusion and erythropoietin; neutropenia by G-CSF or GM-CSF; 5 azacytidine improves blood count; bone marrow transplantation in patients below < 60 years.

ACUTE LEUKEMIA

Essentials of diagnosis

- Fever, bleeding. fatigue of sudden onset, lymphadenopathy, anaemia
- Cytopenia or pancytopenia with more than 20% blasts in marrow and premature cells in peripheral smear.
- Often DIC (promyelocytic leukemia and monocytic leukemia)
- Bleeding takes the form of epistaxis, gingival bleeding (due to thrombocytopenia) and fever is due to gram negative sepsis.
- Sternal tenderness, hepatosplenomegaly; mediastinal mass in T-cell ALL.
- Hypercellular marrow; Auer rod in myeloblasts which are peroxidose positive; monoblasts are butyrate esterase positive; TdT positive for lymphoblasts; CD_5CD_7 positivity for T cell lymphoblasts.

Treatment

- When very high count impairs circulation with headache confusion, dyspnea – emergent leukapheresis with chemotherapy is the answer.

ALL – Induction with vincrystine, prednisolone and L-asparginase, 5-6 cycles followed by CNS radiation and intrathecal methoteaxate.

Consolidation with vincrystine, adriamycin and prednisolone.

Maintenance for 2 years with 6 MP, methotrexate.

AML Induction with daunomycin, cytosar and thioguanine; 5-6 cycles followed by intrathecal cytosar.

Maintenance with alternating DAT and COAP regime for 2 years.

- Bone marrow transplantation (autologous or allogenic) can be undertaken after patient attends remission with induction.
- Chemotherapy plus retinoic acid achieves long term remission in promyelocytic leukemia.

CHRONIC LYMPHOCYTIC LEUKEMIA (CLL)

- Indolent slowly progressive disease with lymphocytosis (> 5000/cmm), mature appearance of lymphocytes which have coexpression of CD_5 and CD_{19} but are immunoincompetent.
- Lymphadenopathy, hepatosplenomegaly; anaemia and thrombocytopenia in stage III and stage IV disease.
- While the systemic disease remains stable, a lymphnode can transform to large cell lymphoma (Richter's syndrome).
- *Treatment* is with fludarabine 25 mg/m² IV for 5 days, every 4-6 weeks for 4-6 cycles; alternatively chlorambucil 0.6-1 mg/kg orally every 3 weeks for 6 months. Both can be combined with rituximab 375 mg/m² IV weekly for 4-8 doses.

Associated autoimmune haemolytic anaemia or immune thrombocytopenia be treated with prednisolone or splenectomy. Bone marrow transplantation is reserved for rare young patients.

Table 9.2: Difference between leukemia and leukemoid reaction

Leukemia	Leukemoid reaction
1. No specific	Inflammatory disease (pneumonia, vasculitis)
2. Neutrophils: Left shift with myeloid cells earlier than bands; WBC > 100,000/uL	Mature neutrophils > 90% and WBC usually < 50,000/uL
3. Leukocyte alkaline phosphatase (LAP) low in CML	Leukocyte alkaline Phosphatase (LAP) high
4. Eosinophilia, basophilia, or monocytosis frequently seen	Not seen
5. Platelets-qualitatively abnormal, large; count > 1,000,000/uL; abnormal aggregation; thrombocytopenia may occur	Platelets-small; not more than 600,000-700,000/uL with normal aggregation
6. Splenomegaly (25-75%)	No splenomegaly
7. Bone marrow-megakaryocytic and platelet clumping; possibly fibrosis	Bone marrow-hyperplastic with normal karyotype
8. Karyotype may be abnormal, esp. in CML with the philadelphia chromosome; bcr-abl by Southern blot or PCR; Clonality by x-linked inactivation techniques	None of these changes are seen

HAIRY CELL LEUKEMIA

- An indolent cancer of B lymphocytes with pancytopenia, massive splenomegaly.
- Bone marrow usually yields dry tap but biopsy shows characteristic hairy cells coexpressing CD_{22} and CD_{11c} and characteristic staining with TRAP.
- Splenic red pulp is infiltrated with hairy cells.

- *Treatment* is with cladribine 0.14 mg/kg/d by IV infusion for 7 days.

NON-HODGKIN'S LYMPHOMA

Essentials of Diagnosis

- Painless lymphadenopathy-isolated or widespread, can be in retroperitoneum, mesentery, pelvis.
- Fever, drenching night sweats or weight loss.
- Involvement of Waldeyer ring.
- Involvement of bone marrow (paratrabecular lymphoid aggregates), meninges.
- Lymphnode biopsy is diagnostic.

Treatment

- *Low grade lymphoma*: radiation for localized disease; CVP (chlorambucil, vincrystine, prednisolone)/ fludarabine for widespread disease. Young patient with aggressive low grade lymphoma may be offered allogenic bone marrow transplantation.
- *Intermediate grade NHL* – for limited disease CHOP regime plus local radiation; for diffuse disease - CHOP regime plus rituximab. Autologous stem cell transplantation in high risk lymphoma.

HODGKIN'S LYMPHOMA

Essentials of Diagnosis

- Painless lymphadenopathy, commonly in neck.
- Often generalised pruritus and B symptoms – fever, night sweat and weight loss
- Pain in the involved node after alcohol ingestion.
- Reed Stersnburg cells in lymphnode and often bone marrow biopsy.

Table 9.3: Clinical differences between Hodgkin's and non-Hodgkin's lymphoma

Hodgkin's disease	Non-Hodgkin's lymphoma
1. Cellular derivation-unresolved	90% B-cell; 10% T-cell
2. Localised to a single group of nodes (cervical, mediastinal, para aortic)	Rarely monocytic Involvement of multiple peripheral nodes
3. Spreads by contiguity	Non contiguous spread
4. Mesenteric nodes and Waldeyer's ring rarely involved	Commonly involved
5. Extranodal involvement-uncommon	Common
6. Bone marrow involvement-Uncommon	Common
7. Chromosomal translocation-yet to be described	Common
8. Curability > 75%	< 30-40%

Treatment

- Radiation for localised disease; ABVD regime for stage IIIB and stage IV disease. When relapse occurs high dose chemotherapy be combined with autologous stem cell transplantation.

MULTIPLE MYELOMA

Essentials of diagnosis

- Bone pain, often in lower back and ribs.
- Replacement of bone marrow by malignant plasma cells.
- Hyperviscosity syndrome – mucosal bleeding, vertigo, visual disturbances, confusion
- Anaemia, pathologic fracture, renal failure, hypercalcemia, fever due to infection.
- Monoclonal paraprotein in serum and urine, light chains in urine.

- ESR is very high but alkaline phosphatase is not raised despite extensive bony involvement.

Treatment

- VAD regime in younger patients; melphalan in elderly followed by autologous stemcell transplantation.
- Thalidomide
- *Treatment* of hypercalcemia and renal failure; pamidronate 90 mg IV monthly reduces pathologic fracture.

WALDENSTROM'S MACROGLOBULINEMIA

- Symptoms of hyperviscosity; splenomegaly is common; ↑ monoclonal IgM paraprotein; hepatosplenomegaly and lymphadenopathy but no bone tenderness.
- Monoclonal IgM in SPEP; bone marrow infiltration with plasmacytic lymphocytes.
- *Treatment* is with plasmapheresis in emergency; chemotherapy with cladribine, cyclophosphamide, chlorambucil, rituximab; autologous stemcell transplantation in younger patients.

IDIOPATHIC THROMBOCYTOPENIC PURPURA (ITP)

- Isolated thrombocytopenia with mucosal or skin bleed (epistaxis, petechiae), purpura, haemorrhagic bullae in mouth.
- No organomegaly, no systemic illness or other abnormality of haematopoietic cell line.
- Normal bone marrow.
- *Treatment* is with prednisolone 1-2 mg/kg/day or high dose IVIg (1 gm/kg) for 1-2 days. Danazol 600 mg per day is another alternative. Non responders or those intolerant to drugs need splenectomy. Immunosuppressive therapy may be required in

occasional patient, often followed by autologous stem cell transplantation. Platelet transfusion is not helpful as transfused platelets do not survive long.

THROMBOTIC THROMBOCYTOPENIC PURPURA (TTP)

- Microangiopathic haemolytic anaemia (fragmented red cells).
- Thrombocytopenia, neurologic and renal abnormalities (confusion, aphasia, headache, renal decompensation).
- Fever, purpura, petechiae, abdominal tenderness (pancreatitis).
- Coagulation tests are normal, Coomb's test is negative.
- *Treatment* is with large volume (80 ml/kg) plasmapheresis till remission. Prednisolone and aspirin can be used in addition to plasmapheresis. Non responders need splenectomy.

HAEMOLYTIC UREMIC SYNDROME (HUS)

- Microangiopathic haemolytic anaemia, thrombocytopenia and renal failure, elevated LDH (due to haemolysis).
- Normal coagulation tests, no neurological abnormality, elevated FDP.
- Endothelial hyaline thrombi in the afferent arterioles and glomeruli in renal biopsy.
- *Treatment* is with high volume plasma pheresis and treatment of renal failure.

VON WILLEBRAND'S DISEASE

- Increased bleeding tendency — epistaxis, gingival bleed, menorrhagia, exacerbated by aspirin.
- Prolonged bleeding time; reduced levels of factor VIII antigen or ristocetin cofactor.

- Reduced level of factor VIII coagulant activity in some.
- Normal platelet number and morphology; platelet aggregation with ADP and collagen are normal
- Desmopression 0.3 µg/kg daily increases vWF by its release from endothelial cells; factor VIII concentrate (now has replaced cryoprecipitate) 20-50 units/kg is also helpful. Both can be supplemented by traxenamic acid 25 mg/kg tid.

DISSEMINATED INTRAVASCULAR COAGULATION

- Microangiopathic haemolytic anaemia.
- Bleeding usually spontaneous from wound or venupuncture site.
- Thrombosis manifesting with digital gangrene, adrenal infarction, renal cortical necrosis.
- Reduced fibrinogen, thrombocytopenia, ↑ FDP in urine, ↑ prothrombin time.
- Recurrent superficial and deep vein thrombosis of cancer is a form of subacute DIC (Trousseau's syndrome).
- *Treatment* is with platelet transfusion, fibrinogen replacement (cryoprecipitate) and replacement of coagulation factors by fresh frozen plasma.
- Heparin 500-750 units per hour IV but antithrombin III level be first raised by fresh frozen plasma.
- EACA 1 gm IV per hour or traxenamic acid 10 mg/kg IV every 8 hours in conjunction with heparin and component transfusions.

10

RHEUMATIC DISORDERS

RHEUMATOID ARTHRITIS

Essentials of diagnosis

- Insidious onset, bilateral symmetrical small joint involvement, progression is centripetal, deformities common (swan neck, boutonniere).
- Prodromal symptoms of malaise, fever, weight loss, morning stiffness.
- X-ray shows juxta articular osteoporosis, joint erosions, narrowing of joint spaces.
- Extraarticular manifestations — subcutaneous nodules, pleuropericarditis, lymphadenopathy, splenomegaly with leukopenia and casculitis (scleritis, aortitis).
- Rheumatoid factor usually positive (IgM against IgG).

Treatment

- Physical and occupational therapy, systemic and articular rest, heat and cold, splint and assistive exercise to preserve joint motion, muscular strength endurance.
- NSAID – particularly Cox 2 inhibitors (Cox 2 is cytokine induced, expressed in inflammatory cells only) particularly valdecoxib 10-20 mg OD, celecoxib 100-200 mg OD, etoricoxib – 30-60 mg daily.
- Disease modifying agents: 1. Penicillamine (rarely used), 2. Gold 10 mg IM first week, 25 mg IM second week. 50 mg weekly IM there after up to maximum of 800 mg, if good response continue till total dose of 1 gm followed by 50 mg IM every 2-4 weeks; alternatively

oral dose is 3 mg twice daily. 3. Hydroxychoroquine 200-400 mg/d. 4. Azathioprine 1mg/kg increased to 3 mg/kg/day.

- TNF inhibitor infliximab.
- Corticosteroids short term to manage pleuro-pericarditis, eye lesions or improve mobility — dose 10 mg PO daily; intra-articular corticosteroids.
- Methotrexate 7.5 mg PO once weekly raised to 15 mg once weekly.
- Leflunomide 100 mg daily for 3 days, then maintenance 20 mg daily.
- Sulfasalazine 0.5 gm twice daily, increased upto 3 gm daily.

SYSTEMIC LUPUS ERYTHEMATOSUS

Essentials of diagnosis

- Occurs mainly in young women.
- Butterfly rash over face (malar).
- Joint symptoms in most patients but deformity is rare and no erosive changes in x-ray.
- Multisystemic involvement due to vasculitis (shrinking lung, nephropathy, coronary, CNS and mesenteric vasculitis)
- Mucous membrane lesions, photosensitivity, nail fold infarct, discoid, lupus, Raynaud's phenomenon, cotton wool retinal spots (cystoid bodies), pleuro-peri carditis, myocarditis, Libman-Sacks endocarditis with valvular regurgitation.
- Lymphadenopathy, splenomegaly, haemolytic anaemia, leucopenia, thrombocytopenia, venous and arterial thrombosis (antiphospholipid syndrome).
- Positive ANA, positive for antibody to native DNA, positive LE cell phenomenon, antibody to SM, false positive VDRL.

Treatment

- Minor joint symptoms treated with NSAID; hydroxy chloroquine upto 400 mg/day.
- Corticosteroids only for serious manifestations like pleuropericarditis, myocarditis, nephritis, convulsion, haemolytic anaemia, thrombocytopenic purpura. CNS disease requires high dose corticosteroid but steroid psychosis may mimic lupus cerebritis.
- Immunosuppressants like cyclophosphamide (particularly for renal disease), chlorambucil, azathioprine for those resistant to corticosteroid.
- Danazol for thrombocytopenia and warfarin for antiphospholipid syndrome.
- High dose cyclophosphamide and prednisolone pulse therapy is particularly helpful in lupus nephritis.

SYSTEMIC SCLEROSIS

Essentials of Diagnosis

- Diffuse thickening of skin (hide bound), telangiectasia, and areas of increased pigmentation and depigmentation.
- Ulceration of finger tips, sclerodactyly, subcutaneous calcification, Raynaud's syndrome.
- Systemic features — dysphagia, GE reflux, pulmonary fibrosis, GI hypomotility, pulmonary vascular disease, pericarditis, heart block, myocardial fibrosis, renal small vessel vasculitis with renal crisis.
- Positive ANA, scleroderma antibody (SCL-70) directed against topoisomerase III may portend grave prognosis.

Treatment

- Usually symptomatic and supportive.
- Calcium channel blockers, losartan for Raynaud's phenomenon.

- Ilioprost, prostacyclin analog for healing of digital ulcers.
- PPI and antacids for GE reflux.
- Prokinetic drugs (cisapride) for GI hypomotility.
- Malabsorption due to bacterial overgrowth is treated with tetracycline 500 mg qid.
- Severe interstitial lung disease is treated with cyclophosphamide but prednisolone has no role.

POLYMYOSITIS – DERMATOMYOSITIS

- Bilateral proximal muscle weakness of legs (difficulty in rising from low chair, climbing stairs) and hands (difficulty in combing).
- In dermatomyositis — heliotrope rash involving malar region and eyelids, periungal erythema, dilatation of nailbed capillaries, scaly patches over dorsum of MCP, chest and back (shawl sign).
- Raised CPK and other muscle enzymes; lymphoid inflammatory infiltrate around muscle fascicles in dermatomyositis and within muscle fiber in polymyositis.
- *Treatment* of both entities is with longterm prednisolone 40-60 mg daily initially; the dose then adjusted downward according to CPK levels. Tumour induced dermatomyositis responds poorly to steroid. IV immunoglobulin is also effective in dermatomyositis resistant to prednisolone.

SJOGREN'S SYNDROME

- 90% of patients are women; the average age is 50 years.
- Dryness of eyes and dry mouth; can occur alone or in association with rheumatoid arthritis or other connective tissue disorders.
- Rheumatoid factor and other autoantibodies are common.
- Increased incidence of lymphoma.

- *Treatment* is symptomatic and supportive with artificial tear, hard candies, sugar free gums, maintenance of good oral hygiene.

POLYARTERITIS NODOSA AND MICROSCOPIC POLYANGITIS

- Classic PAN involves only medium sized vessels, microscopic polyangitis involves small vessels.
- Clinical findings depends upon arteries involved.
- Common symptoms of both include fever and constitutional symptoms, abdominal pain, livido reticularis, mononeuritis multiplex, anaemia, raised ESR.
- Classic PAN is often associated with hypertension but spares the lung vessels, is often associated with HBV and HCV.
- Microscopic polyangitis frequently associated with positive ANCA, pulmonary haemorrhages and glomerulonephritis.
- *Treatment* is with corticosteroid upto 60 mg daily. Critically ill may need IV methylprednisolone 1gm daily for 30 days. Cyclophosphamide is more helpful for microscopic polyangitis either given daily or monthly pulse therapy.
- Diagnosis is by angiography for PAN and biopsy of involved tissue as in microscopic polyangitis.

POLYMYALGIA RHEUMATICA AND GIANT CELL ARTERITIS

- The hall mark of polymyalgia rheumatica is pain and stiffness in shoulder and hips with difficulty in combing, dressing and getting up from low chair.
- In giant cell arteritis there is headache, jaw claudication, visual abnormalities and markedly elevated ESR.
- Low dose prednisolone 10-20 mg daily for few days improves polymyalgia rheumatica but prednisolone

60 mg daily for 1-2 month is needed for giant cell arteritis with gradual tapering as dictated by ESR.

WEGNER'S GRANULOMATOSIS

- Triad of upper respiratory tract disease (sinusitis, mastoiditis, subglottic stenosis), lower respiratory disease, and glomerulonephritis.
- Pathological triad is small vessel vasculities, granulomatous inflammation and necrosis.
- CANCA is relatively sensitive and specific.
- *Treatment* is with cyclophosphamide and prednisolone in severe disease or methotrexate 20 mg weekly for mild disease.

ANKYLOSING SPONDYLITIS

- Chronic low back pain in young adults; progressive limitation of back motion and of chest expansion.
- Transient or permanent peripheral arthritis, uveitis.
- Sclerosis and erosion of sacroiliac joints; ossification of annulus fibrosus, calcification of anterior and lateral spinal ligaments, squaring of vertebra (bamboo spine) in advanced cases.
- High ESR, HLA B-27 positive.
- *Treatment* is with NSAID, but indomethacin 25-50 mg PO daily is most effective, regular exercise program (swimming, prone lying); sulphasalazine for peripheral arthritis (not for spinal or sacroiliac joint disease).

PSORIATIC ARTHRITIS

- Psoriasis precedes arthritis in 80%, arthritis precedes or occurs simultaneously in the rest.
- Arthritis is usually asymmetric with "sausage" appearance of toes and fingers, resembles rheumatoid arthritis but rheumatoid factor is negative.
- Sacroiliac joint involvement is common.

- X-rays shows pencil-in-cup deformity, bony ankylosis, asymmetric sacroilitis and atypical syndesmophytes.
- *Treatment* is symptomatic. NSAID suffice for mild disease. Corticosteroids are less effective. Antimalarials may exacerbate psoriasis. Sulfasalazine and gold may help but methotrexate is definitely beneficial.

REITER'S SYNDROME

- Oligoarthritis, urethritis, conjunctivitis and mouth ulcers.
- Usually follows dysentery or sexually transmitted disease.
- Most patients are HLA-B 27 positive.
- Fever, weight loss, balanitis, keratoderma blenorrhagica, carditis, aortic regurgitation.
- *Treatment* is with NSAID, antibiotics usually tetracycline 250 mg qid for 3 months (enteric Reiter's syndrome does not respond to antibiotics) and sulfasalazine 1 gm bd.

11
ELECTROLYTE DISORDERS

HYPONATREMIA

- Hyponatremia can be hypo/hypervolemic hypotonic hyponatremia or euvolemic hypotonic hyponatremia. Isotonic hyponatremia though less common occurs in hyperlipidemia and hypertonic hyponatremia occurs in hypereglycemia.
- Diarrhoea, vomiting, diuretics, nephropathies, ACE inhibitors cause hypovolemic hypotonic hyponatremia whereas edematous states like CHF, nephrosis cause hypervolemic hypotonic hyponatremia. In SIADH, hypothyroidism, postoperative period and with endurance exercise there is euvolemic hypotonic hyponatremia.
- In SIADH plasma osmolality is low with increased urine osmolality and urine sodium in excess of 20 mEq/L.
- Symptoms in the form of drowsiness, headache, confusion, lack of concentration and delirium appear when serum Na falls below 120 mEq/L
- *Treatment* of asymptomatic SIADH is with water restriction, saline infusion, demeclocycline 300 mg bid, that of symptomatic SIADH is with 3% saline with furosemide with care not to correct plasma osmolality more than 1 mEq/L per hour or 24 mEq/L in first 2 days (for fear of inducing pontine myelinolysis)
- Hypovolemic hypotonic hyponatremia is treated with 0.9% saline or Ringer lactate solutions often complemented by corticosteroids.
- Hypervolemic hyponatremia needs water restriction and diuretics; if CNS symptoms are severe with plasma Na < 110 mEq/L dialysis or 3% NaCl with furosemide may be helpful.

HYPERNATREMIA

- When dehydration is present, orthostatic hypotension and oliguria are typical findings. Hyperthermia, delirium and coma may be seen with severe hyperosmolality.
- *Treatment* is directed towards correcting the cause of fluid loss and replacing water and if needed electrolytes. The reduction of plasma osmolality should not exceed 1 mEq/L/hour for fear of aggravating brain edema due to idiogenic osmoles synthesized in CNS in response to hypernatremia.

HYPOKALEMIA

- Muscular weakness, fatigue, muscle cramps in mild hypokalemia.
- Ileus, hyporeflexia, tetany, hypercapnia, rhabdomyolysis occur in severe hypokalemia.
- ECG – decreased ORS amplitude, broadening of T waves, prominent U waves, depressed ST segment, VPB.
- Oral potassium for mild to moderate deficiency, IV potassium for severe deficiency; rate of infusion not exceeding 40 mEq/L/hr under frequent ECG monitoring to avoid hyperkalemia.

HYPERKALEMIA

- Abdominal distention, muscle weakness, flaccid palsy diarrhoea.
- ECG changes — peaked T waves, widening of QRS, bradycardia, ventricular fibrillation. However, half of patients with serum K^+ above 6.5 mEq/L have normal ECG; hence ECG is not very sensitive.
- *Treatment* is with 1. Calcium gluconate 10% or calcium chloride 5%, 10-30 ml IV; 2. $NaHCO_3$, 44-88 mEq IV; 3. Insulin, 5-10 units IV plus glucose 50%, 50 ml IV; 4. Albuterol 10-20 mg in 4 ml saline nebulized over 10 minutes; 5. Haemo/peritoneal dialysis.

HYPOCALCEMIA

- Cramps, tetany, carpopedal spasm, laryngospasm with stridor, convulsion, cardiac arrhythmia.
- Paresthesia of lips, extremities, abdominal pain.
- Positive: 1. Chvostek's sign (contraction of the facial muscles on taping facial nerve); 2. Trousseau's sign (carpal spasm on occlusion of brachial artery); 3. Tinel's sign.
- Prolonged QT interval in ECG.
- Cataracts and calcification of basal ganglia (in hypoparathyroidism).
- *Treatment* is with (1) calcium gluconate 10-20 ml (10%) IV followed by continuous calcium gluconate infusion, (2) oral calcium and vitamin D supplement, (3) correction of magnesium deficit which by itself will correct hypocalcemia.

Serum calcium falls in the ratio of 0.8-1 mg per 1 gm/ 100 ml fall in plasma albumin; plasma sodium falls 1.6 mEq/L for every 110 mg/dl rise in plasma glucose. Osmolality is 2 Na^+ (mEq/L) + glucose (mg/dL)/18 + BUN (mg/dL)/2.8. Osmoles per kg of water is osmolality, osmoles per litre of solution is osmolarity. 1 mOsm of glucose equals 180 mg/L and 1 mOsm of urea nitrogen equals 28 mg/L.

HYPERCALCEMIA

- Constipation, polyuria.
- Stupor, azotemia and coma is severe hypercalcemia.
- VPB and idioventricular rhythm.
- ECG – shortened QT interval.
- *Treatment* — (1) Emergency treatment with furosemide 40 mg and 3-4 lit/day saline infusion; (2) Bisphosphonates for cancer related hypercalcemia; (3) Calcitonin 4 units/kg intranasal/IM/SC twice daily along with bisphosphonates; (4) IV plicamycin 25 µg/kg/d for 3-4 days; (5) Gallium nitrate 100-200 mg/m^2/d IV for 5 days; (6) Prednisolone.

HYPOPHOSPHATEMIA

- Acute severe hypophosphatemia causes acute haemolytic anaemia, leucocyte and platelet dysfunction; encephalopathy, heart failure; rhabdomyolysis may occur.
- Chronic severe depletion can cause anorexia, pain in muscles and bones and fractures.
- *Treatment* is with oral phosphate supplement or IV phosphorus 620-1240 mg daily.

HYPOMAGNESEMIA

- Weakness, muscle cramps; neuromuscular and CNS hyperirritability with tremor, athetoid movements, nystagmus, positive Babinski sign, confusion, disorientation, tachycardia, hypertension, ventricular arrhythmia.
- *Treatment* is with IV MgSO4 240-1200 mg/day in severe deficit or 200-800 mg/day in 4 divided doses in moderate deficit to keep plasma level around 2.5 mmol/L. K^+ and Ca^{++} may be required as well. MgO 250-500 mg orally 2-4 times daily is useful in chronic hypomagnesemia. Hypokalemia and hypo calcemia of hypomagnesemia do not recover without magnesium supplement.

HYPERMAGNESEMIA

- Muscle weakness, decreased tendon reflexes, confusion progressing to flaccid muscle palsy and even respiratory muscle palsy and cardiac arrest.
- *Treatment* is that of renal failure (most common cause of elevated Mg^{++}). Calcium 100 mg/min IV upto 500 mg acts as antagonist to magnesium. Haemo/peritoneal dialysis may be required.

RESPIRATORY ACIDOSIS

- Confusion, asterixis, myoclonus, somnolence, confusion and coma from carbon dioxide narcosis.

- Increased cerebral blood flow with raised ICP causing headache, papilledema.
- *Treatment* is that of underlying disorder (acute respiratory failure) with mechanical ventilation or reversing the narcotic overdose by naloxone 0.04-2 mg IV.

RESPIRATORY ALKALOSIS

- Anxiety, light headedness, paresthesia, numbness, tingling.
- Tetany.
- *Treatment* is that of cause. Rebreathing into a paper bag increases PCO_2.

Rapid correction of chronic respiratory acidosis can cause posthypercapnic metabolic alkalosis (due to renal lag of bicarbonate excretion); rapid correction of chronic respiratory alkalosis can cause metabolic acidosis.

METABOLIC ACIDOSIS

- Symptoms are those of underlying disorder; can be of increased anion gap (lactic acidosis, diabetic ketoacidosis, alcoholic ketoacidosis, salicylate poisoning, methanol (formic acid), ethylene glycol (oxalic acid), 2. Normal anion gap (diarrhoea, vomiting, RTA).
- *Treatment* is that of underlying disorder, use of large amount of bicarbonates can cause hypernatremia and hyperosmolality; the bicarbonate is converted to CO_2 which enters the cells and worsens intracellular acidosis. Alkali therapy increases phosphofructokinase activity and increases lactate production, aggravating lactic acidosis.

Bicarbonate deficit = 0.5 × kg body wt × (24 − HCO_3^-)

In RTA, bicarbonate supplementation is necessary.

METABOLIC ALKALOSIS

- Metabolic alkalosis is generally associated with hypokalemia and extracellular volume contraction. Symptoms may be orthostatic hypotension, weakness and hyporeflexia.
- Treatment is with 0.9% NaCl, in emergent cases HCl 0.1 Mol/L IV infusion can be undertaken.
- Metabolic alkalosis of primary aldosteronism needs potassium repletion.

12

SKIN DISEASES

ATOPIC DERMATITIS (ECZEMA)

- Pruritic, exudative or lichenified eruption on face, neck, upper trunk, wrists and hands and in antecubital and popliteal folds.
- Personal or family history of allergy (asthma, allergic rhinitis, atopic dermatitis).
- *Treatment* is (1) aluminium subacetate or saline soaks for weeping lesions along with steroid lotions and gels; (2) high to highest potency steroid, ointment for dry lichenified lesions often supplemented with tar preparation. Tacrolimus ointment 0.03-0.1% is the steroid sparing agent. 5% doxepin cream also reduces pruritus, Oral steroid 40-60 mg daily is needed in extensive and more severe disease.
- Eczema herpeticum, a generalised HSV infection with monomorphic vesicles, crusts and erosions superimposed on atopic dermatitis needs oral acyclovir 200 mg 5 times daily or IV acyclovir 10 mg/kg 8 hourly.

LICHEN SIMPLEX (NEURODERMATITIS)

- Chronic itching
- Lichenified (rectangular pigmented) lesions with exaggerated skin lines overlying a thickened well circumscribed scaly plaque.
- Predilection for nape of neck, wrists, forearm, lower leg, popliteal and antecubital areas.
- *Treatment* is with high-highest potent topical steroid, else local injection of triamcinolone acetonide into the lesion.

LICHEN PLANUS

- Pruritic violaceous flat topped papules with fine white streaks and symmetric distribution.
- Lacy white lesions in buccal mucosa, vagina.
- Commonly seen along linear scratch marks (Koebner phenomenon), on anterior wrist, penis and legs.
- Can be seen in GI tract, bladder, larynx.
- Squamous cell carcinoma may develop on lichen simplex lesions.
- *Treatment* is with topical steroid to skin lesions, tretinoin 0.05% cream to mucosal lesions. Topical tacrolimus is effective for oral/vaginal erosive lichen planus.
- Severe cases may require isotretinum, acitretin PO and often PUVA therapy.

PSORIASIS

- Silvery scales on bright red well demarcated plaques.
- Usually in the knees, elbows and scalp.
- Pitting of nails and onycholysis.
- Mild itching (usually).
- Often associated with psoriatic arthropathy.
- *Treatment* is with topical highest potency steroid, along with tar preparation, topical anthralin, 0.05% calcipotriene, topical retinoid (tazarotene gel – 0.05-0.1%). Scalp psoriasis needs tar shampoo daily and steroid topically.
- Extensive psoriasis involving more than 30% of body surface needs (1) UVB or coal tar application with UVB exposure; (2) psoralen plus UVA (PUVA); (3) methotrexate 10-25 mg weekly; (4) acitretin 0.5-1 mg per kg PO daily; (5) thioguanine 40-80 mg PO 2-7 days per week; (6) cyclosporine; (7) sulfasalalazin 1 gm tid.

PITYRIASIS ROSEA

- Oval fawn-coloured scaly eruption following cleavage lines of trunk (Christmas tree pattern). The centres of lesions have crinkled or cigarette paper appearance and a collarette scale.

- Mild pruritus; herald patch precedes eruption by 1-2 weeks.
- *Treatment* is with (1) UVB, (2) prednisolone orally, (3) topical steroids, or (4) erythromycin PO for 2 weeks.

SEBORRHEIC DERMATITIS

- Affects scalp, central face, presternal area, eyelid margins, chest, body folds.
- Oily yellowish scurf or dry scales and underlying erythema.
- *Treatment* (1) Scalp lesion – ketoconazole shampoo 1-2% twice weekly; (2) facial lesion – hydrocortisone 1% oint, desonide or alclometasone ointment along with ketoconazole oint; (3) intertriginous areas – low potency steroid lotions or creams.

TINEA CORPORIS

- Ring-shaped itchy lesion with advancing scaly border with central clearing or scaly patches with a distinct border.
- Hyphae demonstrated in the scraping.
- *Treatment* (1) Topical miconazole 2%, clotrimazole 1%, haloprogin-, econazole 1%, ketoconazole 2%, sulconazole 1%, tolnaftate 1%, oxyconazole 1%, ciclopirox 1%, naftifine 1%, butenafine/terbinafine 1%; (2) systemic – (a) griseofulvin 250-500 mg PO daily for 2-4 weeks, (b) terbenafine 250 mg daily for 1 month, (c) itraconazole 200 mg daily for 7 days.

TINEA VERSICOLOR

- Pale macules with fine scales or hyperpigmented macules.
- Velvety, pink, whitish or brown macules that scale with scraping.

- Central upper trunk the most frequent site.
- Yeast and short hyphae on microscopic examination of scales.
- *Treatment* (1) Topical – (a) selenium sulfide application for 5-15 minutes daily for 7 days, (b) ketoconazole shampoo for 5 minutes weekly for maintenance of remission, (c) sodium thiosulphate lotion, (d) zinc-pyrithrone shampoo or sulphur – salicylic acid soap for prophylaxis. (2) Systemic – ketoconazole 400 mg single dose or 200 mg daily for 7 days; patient advised not to take bath for 12-18 hours because it is delivered to skin by sweat.

DISCOID LUPUS ERYTHEMATOSUS

- Localised red papules, usually on the face.
- Scaling, follicular plugging, atrophy, dyspigmentation and telangiectasia of involved areas.
- *Treatment* (1) Topical—(a) highly potent corticosteroid oint, (b) Local infiltration with triamcinolone; (2) systemic (a) hydroxy chloroquine or quinacrine 100 mg daily, (b) isotretinoin 1 mg/kg/day, (c) thalidomide 50-100 mg daily.

MYCOSIS FUNGOIDES (CUTANEOUS T CELL LYMPHOMA)

- Localised or generalised erythematous scaling plaques.
- Lymphadenopathy, pruritus.
- Circulating Sezary cells; biopsy confirmatory.
- *Treatment* (1) Topical mechlorethamine, steroids; (2) systemic – retinoids, alpha intereferon; (3) PUVA and radiation therapy.

POMPHOLYX

- 'Tapioca' vesicles of 1-2 mm on palms and soles and sides of fingers, associated with pruritus.
- Vesicles may coalesce to form multiloculated blisters.

- Scaling and fissuring may follow drying of blisters.
- Appearance in third decade with life long recurrences.
- *Treatment* is with topical high potent steroid, wearing of cotton globes, avoidance of nickel; PUVA therapy to hands.

DERMATOPHYTID

- Pruritic, grouped vesicular lesions involving the sides and flexor aspects of the fingers and palms.
- Fungal infection elsewhere in the body but no fungus demonstrated in lesion.
- *Treatment* is oral antifungal and topical antifungal of primary lesion.

PORPHYRIA CUTANEA TARDA

- Non-inflammatory painless blisters on sunexposed areas, especially dorsal surface of hands.
- Hypertrichosis and hyperpigmentation of face.
- Elevated urine porphyrins.
- *Treatment* is stoppage of all triggering medications (estrogen), stopping of alcohol consumption, low dose antimalarial (hydroxychloroquine 200 mg twice weekly), phlebotomy.

IMPETIGO

- Of two types (1) Vesiculopustular type with thick golden crusted lesions caused by Strepto or Staphylococcus; (2) bullous lesion caused by Strepto or Staphylococcus; (3) bullous lesion caused by *Staph aureus*.
- Ecthyma is a deeper form of impetigo with ulceration and scarring.
- *Treatment* is with (1) erythromycin/cloxacillin orally with local mupirocin oint. Recurrent impetigo is associated with nasal carriage of *S. aureus*, treated with rifampicin 600 mg daily for 5 days or intranasal mupirocin twice daily for 5 days.

ALLERGIC CONTACT DERMATITIS

- Erythema and edema, with pruritus, often followed by vesicles and bullae in the area of contact.
- Later weeping, crusting and secondary infection.
- Patch test with agent usually positive.
- Most common agents are soaps, detergents, hair dyes, preservatives, latex.
- Weeping and crusting are typically due to allergic and not irritant dermatitis.
- *Treatment* is with (1) calamine lotion, potent steroid gel/cream; (2) systemic steroid for 3 weeks in full dosage.

ACNE VULGARIS

- Occurs often at puberty, though onset may be delayed into the third or fourth decade.
- Open and closed comedones over face, neck, upper chest, back.
- Severity varies from purely comedonal acne to cysts or nodules.
- In ladies and girls exclude hyperandrogenism due to polycystic ovary.
- *Treatment* (1) *comedonal acne* — (a) tretinoin 0.025% cream at night, 2 times weekly to daily, (b) tazarotene gel as used in psoriasis, (c) benzoxl peroxide 2.5-10%, (d) erythromycin or minocycline; (2) *Papular inflammatory acne* — (a) topical antibiotic (erythromycin, clindamycin), (b) oral minocycline 50-100 mg bid, (c) oral contraceptives or spironolactone 50-100 mg daily as antiandrogen; (3) *Severe acne* — isotretinoin 0.5-1 mg/kg/day PO for 20 weeks or total dose of 120 mg/kg; (4) intralesional triamcinolone; (5) laser, dermabrasion.

ROSACEA

- Has three components (a) vascular component with erythema and telangiectasia; (b) acneform component; (c) glandular component with rhinophyma

- *Treatment* is with mid potency steroid lotion or cream (not ointment) twice daily application.

MUCOCUTANEOUS CANDIDIASIS

- Severe pruritus of vulva, anus, body folds.
- Superficial denuded beefy red areas with or without satellite vesicopustules.
- Whitish curd like concretions on oral and vaginal mucosa.
- Yeast on microscopic examination of scales or curd.
- *Treatment* (1) Nail and skin— cliclopirox cream, nystatin cream, miconazole, econazole, ketocanazole cream, gentian violet 1%; (2) vulvar/vaginal — miconazole oint/clotrimazole suppository/nistatin tab locally; resistant cases need ketoconazole 200 mg bid for 5 days or fluconazole 150 mg once PO.

ERYTHEMA MULTIFORME

- Symmetric erythematous skin lesion, recurrent
- May be macular, papular, urticarial, bullous or purpuric
- Erythema multiforme major is Stevens Johnson syndrome and favours trunk but erythema multiforme minor favours extensor surfaces, palms, soles or mucous membrane.
- Mycoplasma infection, NSAID, phenytoin, sulfa can cause Stevens Johnson syndrome; HSV infection – erythema multiforme minor.
- *Treatment* is (1) high dose corticosteroid 100-250 mg daily before blistering occurs; (2) IV Ig 0.75 g/kg/day for 4 days; (3) antistaphyloccal antibiotics for prevention of secondary infection.

ERYSIPELAS

- Edematous, spreading, circumscribed erythematous area with or without vesicles and bullae.
- Pain, chills, fever and systemic toxicity.

- Central face frequently involved.
- *Treatment* is with anti Strepto – Staphylococcal antibiotic, i.e. dicloxacillin, erythromycin, azithro/roxithromycin, cephalosporin but not quinolones.

PEMPHIGUS

- Relapsing crops of bullae, often preceded by mucous membrane bullae, erosions and ulcerations.
- Positive Nikolsky's sign (extension of bulla on pressure).
- Acantholysis on biopsy; immune fluorescein studies are confirmatory – IgG mg C_3 in epidermis.
- Can be (1) pemphigus vulgaris or its variant pemphigus vegetans; (2) more superficially blistering pemphigus foliaceus and its variant pemphigus erythematosus.
- Secondary infection commonly occurs and is the major cause of morbidity and mortality.
- *Treatment* is (1) high dose prednisolone 80-360 mg daily along with immunosuppressants, i.e. azathioprine 100-150 mg daily/methotrexate 25 mg weekly/mycophenolate mofetil 1 gm twice daily; (2) Adjunctive measures – tetracycline 500 mg QID with nicotinamide 500 mg bid, dapsone 25-100 mg daily; sodium thiomalate; (3) IVIg or pulse IV cyclophosphamide in refractory cases.

BULLOUS PEMPHIGOID

- Tense blisters in flexural areas in elderly with remission and exacerbation; oral lesions in one-third.
- IgG and C_3 deposit in dermo-epidermal junction in biopsy.
- *Treatment* is as for pemphigus.

DERMATITIS HERPETIFORMIS

- Pruritic papules, vesicles and papulo vesicles mainly on elbows, knees, buttocks, posterior neck and scalp.
- Circulating endomysium antibodies in all cases; granular IgA deposit along dermal papillae.

- Associated gluten sensitive enteropathy (mostly subclinical).
- Increased risk of developing lymphoma.
- *Treatment* is with gluten free diet, dapsone 100-200 mg/day.

SCABIES

- Pruritic vesicles and pustules in "runs" or "galleries" on finger webs, and the heels of the palms and in wrist creases.
- Red papules or nodules on the scrotum, shaft or glans penis are pathognomonic.
- Mites, ova and brown dots of feces visible microscopically.
- *Treatment* is with (1) GBHC 1% lotion/cream overnight, (2) permethrin 5% cream single application, (3) crotamiton cream/lotion for 4 nights, (4) GBHC application 20-35%, (5) ivermectin single oral dose 200 µg/kg, (6) treatment of associated pyoderma with antibiotics, (7) treatment of pruritic postscabetic papules with high potency steroid ointments, (8) disinfection of clothing.

PEDICULOSIS

- Pruritus with excoriation.
- Nits on hair shafts, lice on skin or clothes.
- "Sky blue" macules on inner thighs or lower abdomen in pubic louse infestation.
- *Treatment* is (1) GBHC lotion or cream, (2) permethrin 5% cream for body louse and 1% rinse for head louse, (3) malathion 1% lotion.

ERYTHEMA NODOSUM

- Painful red nodules without ulceration on anterior aspect of legs.
- Slow regression over several weeks to resemble contusion.

- Associated with various infections — tuberculosis, syphilis, IBD, oral contraceptive, deep mycosis.
- *Treatment* is (1) that of primary cause, (2) NSAID, (3) saturated solution of pot. iodide, (4) corticosteroids orally.

ALOPECIA

- Cicatriccal baldness follows lichen planopilaris, chronic DSE, scleroderma, fungal infection of scalp.
- Nonscarring alopecia follows iron deficiency, hypothyroidism.
- Androgenic pattern baldness in male needs 5% minoxidill twice daily application along with finasteride 1 mg daily orally (only in male).
- Thinning of hair in female is equivalent to androgenic male baldness and is treated with minoxidil 5%.
- Alopecia areata involves beard, brows, scalp, with well demarcated areas without scarring. Exclamation hairs may be seen.
- *Treatment* is (1) intralesional triamcinolone 2.5-10 mg/ml injected in aliquots of 0.1 ml at 1-2 cm interval, (2) anthralin 0.5% oint daily, (3) topical diphencyprone and squaric acid dibutylester.

ONYCHOMYCOSIS

- Lusterless, brittle, hypertrophic nails.
- Hyphae seen in ko preparation of nail or PAS staining of histologic section of nail plate.
- *Treatment* (1) Topical – (a) naftifine gel 1% or ciclopirox nail lacquer 8% applied twice daily for 4-6 months for finger nails and 12-18 months for toe nails – indicated for minimally thickened nails; (2) systemic – (a) griseofulvin 750 mg or more daily for six months, (b) itraconazole 200 mg daily for 3 months, (c) terbinafine 250 mg daily for 6 weeks are indicated for finger nails. Toe nails are resistant with low success rate even with prolonged therapy.

13

POISONING

Poisoning can present with coma, convulsion, hypothermia hypotension, hypertension, arrhythmia, hyperthermia, etc.

COMA

- Associated with ingestion of alcohol, opioids, phenothiazines, antidepressants, barbiturates, benzodiazepines which may lead to respiratory failure abruptly or due to aspiration of gastric contents. Hypoxia and hypoventilation may aggravate arrhythmia, hypotension and seizures.
- *Emergency management* of coma is (1) establishing patent airway by positioning, suction, oropharyngeal airway (2) supplemental oxygen/ventilatory support, (3) maintenance of adequate circulation to prevent renal shut down, (4) Drugs — (a) 50% dextrose 50–100 ml IV, thiamine 100 mg IM to take care of hypoglycemia, (b) naloxone 0.4–2 mg IV for opioid over dose or else longer acting nalmefene (c) flumazenil 0.2–0.5 mg IV repeated every half minute to a maximum of 3 mg for benzodiazepine overdose.

HYPOTHERMIA

- Commonly accompanies coma due to alcohol, opioid, barbiturates, benzodiazepine,
- *Treatment* is external rewarming for mild to moderate hypothermia (30°–36°C) and active internal rewarming by warm IV fluids (43°C), warm humid O_2 (42°–46°C), peritoneal lavage (KCl-free fluid), esophageal rewarming tubes.

HYPOTENSION

- Cyanides, CO, arsenic, barbiturates, TCA cause hypotension so also betablockers, calcium channel blockers.
- *Treatment* is (a) IV fluids along with dopamine 5–15 mg/kg/min infusion. Norepinephrine is preferred over dopamine in TCA induced hypotension, (b) glucagon 5–10 mg IV for betablocker poisoning, (c) calcium chloride 20 mg/kg IV for calcium channel blockers overdose.

CONVULSION

- Antihistamines, amphetamine, cocaine, lindane, PCP, TCA, organophosphorus can cause convulsion so also hypoxia, hypoglycemia, alcohol withdrawal, electrolyte abnormalities, CNS infection, etc.
- *Treatment* is with lorazepam 2 mg IV over 2 minutes, or midazolam 5–10 mg IM. If convulsion continues or recurs give phenytoin, or phenobarb 15 mg/kg IV over 30 minutes followed by IV maintenance with phenytoin.

ARRHYTHMIAS

- Besides poisons, they can be due to hypoxia, metabolic acidosis, electrolyte imbalance.
- For tachyarrhythmias induced by chlorinated solvents, sympathomimetics give propranolol 1–5 mg IV or esmolol 25–100 µg/kg/min IV. For TCA induced tachyarrhythmias sodium bicarbonate 500–100 mEq IV is essential.

GENERAL PRINCIPLES OF TREATMENT IN POISONING

1. Gastrointestinal decontamination
   (a) Induction of emesis in conscious cooperative patients by giving concentrated salt solution, stimulation of pharyngeal wall, syrup ipecac 30 ml, in a glass of water.
   (b) Gastric lavage when emesis is refused, unsuccessful or contraindicated.

(c) Activated charcoal absorbs most drugs and poisons except cyanide and alcohol. Dose 60–100 gm
(d) Catharsis – Mg SO$_4$ 10% 2–3 ml/kg or Sorbitol 70% 1–2 ml/kg.
2. Dialysis. Haemodialysis for methanol, salicyclate; charcoal haemoperfusion for phenobarbitone

Antidotes

Acetaminophen	Acetylcysteine
Anticholinengics	Physostigmine
Organophosphates	Atropine and pralidoxime
Benzodiazapine	Flumazenil
Carbon monoxide	Oxygen
Cyanide	Sodium nitrite, sodium thiosulfate
Digitalis	Digoxin specific fab antibodies
Heavy metals	Specific chelating agents
Methanol and ethylene glycol	Ethyl alcohol and fomepizole
Opioids	Naloxone, nalmefene

Acids and Corrosives

- Do not induce emesis, give plenty of milk and water, remove remaining corrosive by careful gastric lavage; do esophagoscopy carefully to assess extent of damage.
- Alkalis with pH above 12 cause deeply penetrating necrosis.

Arsenic

- Abdominal pain, diarrhoea, vomiting, muscle cramp.
- *Treatment* is gastric lavage, activated charcoal, prompt rehydration, dimer caprol 10%, 3–5 mg/kg IM every 6 hours for 2 days followed by penicillamine 100 mg/kg/d

in 4 divided doses or DMSA 10 mg/kg every 8 hours for 1 week.

Atropine and belladonna

- Dryness of mouth, difficulty in swallowing, thirst, blurred vision, dilated pupils, tachycardia, fever, delirium, myoclonus.
- *Treatment* is with (a) physostigmine 1 mg IV over 5 minutes under ECG monitoring for emergency, (b) gastric lavage, activated charcoal, (c) sedation for convulsion, (d) control of hyperthermia.

Carbon Monoxide

- Severe headache, confusion, syncope, hypotension, seizure, coma
- Flushed face (cherry red)
- *Treatment* is with 100%. O_2 through face mask/endotracheal tube and hyperbaric oxygen.

Cyanide

- Odor of bitter almond in patient's breath or vomitus
- High venous oxygen saturation
- *Treatment* is (a) gastric lavage, activated charcoal, (2) amylnitrate inhalation followed by sodium nitrate 6 mg/kg IV and then sodium thiosulphate 250 mg/kg IV.

Ethyl alcohol

- Euphoria, ataxia, stupor, coma, respiratory arrest
- *Treatment* is gastric lavage and activated charcoal, 50% dextrose 50 ml followed by 10% DW with insulin and vit B_1 to accelerate alcohol metabolism.

Methanol and ethylene glycol

- Toxicity is due metabolism of methanol to formic acid, and ethylene glycol to glycolic and oxalic acid.

- After several hours of ingestion – high anion gap metabolic acidosis, convulsion, coma, tachypnoea and renal failure (in ethylene glycol only).
- *Treatment* (a) severe toxicity – haemodialysis, (b) Mild toxicity – ethanol 5–10%, 50 gm IV or fomepizole.

Opioids

- Mild intoxication – euphoria, drowsiness, constricted pupils
- Severe intoxication – hypotension, hypothermia, coma, respiratory arrest.
- Propoxyphene, tramadol, dextromethorpnan and meperidine cause seizure.
- Heroin effect lasts for 3 hours but methadone effect for 48–72 hours.
- *Treatment* is naloxone 0.4–2 mg IV; upto 10–20 mg IV for propoxyphene, codeine and fentanyl.

Organophosphates and carbamates

- Abdominal cramp, diarrhoea, vomiting, salivation, lacrimation, miosis, seizure, muscle palsy, excessive bronchial secretion, wheezing
- Symptoms and signs of poisoning may persist or recur over several days, especially with highly lipid soluble agents like fenothion.
- *Treatment* is with (a) atropine 2 mg IV every 5 minutes till mouth is dry and pupil is dilated, (b) pralidoxime 1–2 gm IV and then 200–400 mg/hr infusion (only effective for organophosphorus).

Salicylates

- Moderate intoxication – deep and rapid breathing, tachycardia, tinnitus, high anion gap acidosis.
- Serious intoxication – agitation, confusion, coma, seizure, pulmonary edema, hyperthermia.
- Blood examination — high salicylate level, ↑ anion gap metabolic acidosis with respiratory alkalosis.

- *Treatment* (a) stomach wash, activated charcoal (ratio of activated charcoal to aspirin is 10:1), (b) IV sodium bicarbnate, (c) alkaline diuresis by saline infusion with $NaHCO_3$ (d) haemodialysis (salicylate level above 100 mg/dl).

Snake bite

- Poison is neurotoxic (coral snake, cobra); cytolytic (rattle snake, pit vipers).
- Neurotoxic envenomation – ptosis, dysphagia, diplopia, respiratory arrest.
- Cytolytic venom — tissue destruction, haemorrhage, haemolysis.
- *Treatment* (a) immobilize the patient, (b) ice application, tourniquet, incision and suction less dependable, (c) antivenin treatment.

14

PSYCHIATRIC DISORDERS

ANXIETY DISORDERS

Generalised anxiety

- Somatic symptoms referable to autonomic nervous system – dry mouth, tachycardia, sweating, restlessness, dyspnoea, paresthesias, insomnia, lack of concentration, tremor, apprehension, headache, hyperactivity, near syncope.

Panic disorder

- Unpredictable episodes of short-lived intense anxiety with marked distressing physiologic manifestations with feeling of impending doom, choking, smothering.

Obsessive compulsive disorders

- Intrusion of irrational idea or emotion forcing patient to act or think irrationally, Completion of the act alleviates the anxiety, e.g. repeated hand washing, checking for door bolts.

Phobic disorders

- A form of displacement in which patients transfer feelings of anxiety from their true object to one that can be avoided.

Dissociative disorders

- Fugue (sudden unexpected travel away from home with inability to recall), amnesia, somnambulism, belong to this class which are precipitated by emotional crisis and resemble temporal lobe dysfunction.

Treatment

A. Benzodiazepines are anxiolytics. The doses are—
alprazolam 0.5–4 mg daily, chlordiazepoxide 10–100
mg daily, diazepam 5–30 mg daily, lorazepam 2–4 mg
daily, oxazepam 10–60 mg daily. Buspirone 10–60 mg
daily is antianxiety as well as antidepressant.
   • Hypnotic agents by promoting sleep remove anxiety.
     Their doses are estazolam 1–2 mg, flurazepam 15–
     30 mg, quazepam 7.5–15 mg, temazepam, 15–30 mg,
     triazolam – 0.125–0.25 mg, zolpidem 5–10 mg and
     zaleplon 5–10 mg. Propranolol 20–40 mg takes care
     of adrenergic symptoms of anxiety.
   • Diazepam and chlordiazepoxide have very long half
     life (> 20 hours), where as triazolam and zolpidem
     have short half life of 1–5 hours and zaleplon – very
     short half life of 1 hour.
B. Panic attack is terminated by sublingual lorazepam
   or alprazolam but for prolonged treatment SSRI like
   setraline 25–50 mg/day augmented with lithium may
   be used.
C. Phobias are treated with SSRI (paroxetine, setraline,
   fluvoxamine) or with gabapentine.
D. Obsessive compulsive disorder responds to SSRI,
   clomipramine, fluoxetine, buspirone, etc.

SOMATOFORM DISORDERS

• Subjective complaints far exceed objective findings.
• Physical symptoms refer to one or more organ systems
  and are not intentional.
• Correlations of symptoms development and psychologic
  stress.
• Can take the form of (1) conversion disorder – like apho-
  nia, paralysis, pseudoepileptic seizure; (2) somatisation
  disorder with multiple complaints referable to several
  organ systems; (3) hypochondriasis (fear and preoccu-
  pation of disease); (4) somatoform pain disorder.

Treatment is mainly by psychologic, behavioral and social approach rather than medicine.

PSYCHOTIC DISORDERS

- Can be (1) schizophrenic disorders comprising (a) hebephrenia marked by incoherent and incongruous affect, (b) catatonic — rigidity and mutism or alternation between excitement and stupor, (c) paranoid — persecutory or grandiose delusions with hallucinations; (2) delusional disorders with minimal impairment of daily activities; (3) schizo affective disorders; (4) schizophreniform disorders (duration of illness < 6 months).
- Symptoms and signs — (a) bizarre appearance, unkempt blandness, reduced motor activity but can have catatonic stupor and excitement, (b) social withdrawal, (c) verbal utterances, neologism, echolalia, verbigeration, (d) flat affect, (e) delusional fantasy (paranoid thinking) and adoptive counter measures, (f) auditory hallucinations (visual hallucination is common with organic brain syndromes).

Table 14.1: Differences between psychosis and neurosis

	Psychosis	Neurosis
Etiology		
Biological factors	More important	Less important
Environmental factors	Less important except in reactive psychosis	More important
Psychopathology		
Personality disintegration	Severe	Partial
Clinical Manifestations		
1. Touch with reality	Lost	Not lost
2. Insight into the illness	Lost (Patient believes that he is all right)	Not lost (Patient complains of illness)

	Psychosis	Neurosis
3. Judgement (i.e. capacity to discriminate between right and wrong, good and bad, ethical and unethical).	Lost	Not Lost
4. Social relationship and behaviour	Affected	Not affected
5. Personal hygiene.	Neglected	Not neglected
6. Distrurbances of mental functions like thinking, emotion and behaviour.	Gross	Minor
7. Disturbances of intelligence, memory, attention, consciousness and orientation.	Common in organic psychosis	Rare
8. Disturbances of thought (viz. delusions) and perception (viz. illusions and hallucinations)	Common	Rare
Course and prognosis.	More malignant than benign Difficult to treat. Recovery may not be always possible or complete. Relapses are common.	More benign than malignant Easier to treat, Recovery possible and sometimes complete. Relapses are common.

Treatment

Hospitalization if patient's behaviour shows gross disorganization.

1. Oral neuroleptic medications—chlorpromazine 100–4000 mg daily, thioridazine 100–600 mg daily, misoridazine 50–400 mg daily, perphenazine 16–64 mg daily, trifluperazine 5–60 mg daily, flufenazine

2–60 mg daily, loxapine 20–200 mg daily, clozapine 200–900 mg daily, haloperiodol 2–60 mg daily, risperidone 2–10 mg daily, olanzapine 5–10 mg daily, quetiapine 200–800 mg daily. Maximum anticholinergic side effects (dry mouth, visual blurring, palpitation) are with chlorpromazine, thioridazine, clozapine and maximum extrapyramidal effects are with perphenazine, trifluperazine, flufenazine, thiothixene, haloperidol, loxapine (in the form of tardive dyskinesia, akathisia and even acute dystonia). Concurrent antiparkinsonian medication like trihexy phenidyl 2–5 mg tid, benztropine mesylate 1–2 mg tid or amantadine 100 mg tid be prescribed.

2. Antidepressants may be used in conjunction with neuroleptics if significant depression is present. Resistant cases may require concomitant use of lithium, carbamazepine or valproic acid. Lorazepam 1–2 mg daily may be added to treat an agitated or catatonic patient.

3. Antipsychotic drug overdose (haloperidol, flufenazine) can cause catatonic syndrome, often misdiagnosed as catatonic schizophrenia and inappropriately treated with more antipsychotic drugs.

4. Injectable neuropleptics weekly of monthly for maintenance once acute symptoms subside

5. ECT for highly agitated patients/depressed patients.

Symptoms that are ameliorated by these drugs include hyperactivity, hostility, aggression, delusions, halucinations, irritability and poor sleep. Negative symptoms like social withdrawal, psychomotor retardation and poor interpersonal relations only improve with atypical antipsychotics (clozapine, risperidone, olanzapine, quetiapine, ziprasidone) but they also in increase QTC with possible risk of arrhythmia.

Neuroleptic malignant syndrome (NMS) is a catatonia-like state manifested by extrapyramidal signs, hyperpyrexia, muscle rigidity, diaphoresis, confusion and coma. *Treatment* is with IV fluids, dantrolene 50 mg IV, bromocriptine 2.5–10 mg tid PO, amantadine 100 mg bid, clozapine and in resistant cases ECT.

DEPRESSION

- Lowered mood, varying from mild sadness to intense feeling of guilt, worthlessness and hopelessness.
- Difficulty in thinking, lack of concentration, indecisiveness, rumination.
- Loss of interest, withdrawal from work and recreation
- Somatic complaints like headache, sleep disturbance, fatigue, anorexia, poor libido.
- Severe depression- delusions of a hypochondriacal or persecutory nature, suicidal ideation.
- *Treatment* is with (1) ECT for severely depressed with suicidal tendency. (2) TCA-amitriptyline 150–300 mg daily, amoxapine 150–400 mg daily, clomipramine 100–250 mg daily, desipramine 100–300 mg daily, doxepine 150–300 mg daily, imipramine 150–300 mg daily, maprotiline 100–300 mg daily, nortriptyline 100–150 mg daily, protriptyline 15–60 mg daily, trazodone 100–400 mg daily, trimipramine 75–200 mg daily, buproprion 300–450 mg daily. (3) MAO inhibitors – phenelzine 45–90 mg daily, tranylcypromine 20–50 mg daily. (4) SSRI and others – fluoxetine 20–80 mg daily, fluvoxamine 100–300 mg daily, paroxetine 20–50 mg daily, setraline 50–200 mg daily, venlafaxine 150–225 mg daily, mirtazapin 15–45 mg daily, citalopram 20–40 mg daily. The medication be continued for 6–12 months and then gradually tapered over months. Antidepressants should be continued indefinitely at full dosage in people with more that 2 episodes after age 40 or one episode after age 50 and first episode before age of 20 years. (5) Adjunctive therapy includes (a) lithium 600–900 mg/day, (b) levothyroxine 25 µg daily,

(c) dextroamphetamine 5–30 mg/d, (d) methylphenidate 10–45 mg/d. (6) Transcranial magnetic stimulation and vagal nerve stimulation are effective in resistant nonpsychotic depression.

Most TCA be given as single dose at bedtime starting at a lower dose with gradual build up. A full trial consists of giving maximum daily dose for 6 weeks. Therapeutic plasma level are nortriptyline 50–150 ng/ml, imipramine 200–250 ng/ml, desipramine 100–250 ng/ml. Withdrawal symptoms like agitation, dysphoric mood occur with SSRI withdrawal. Psychotic depression be treated with antipsychotic, e.g. perphenazine with SSRI.

Table 14.2: Difference between endogenous and neurotic depression

Endogenous depression	Neurotic depression
1. Significant stress situation preceding the attack absent or of a minor intensity.	1. Significant stress situation preceding the attack always present and is of moderate or severe intensity.
2. Biological factors like heredity, constitution, etc. are more important than the environmental factors as etiological agents.	2. Environmental factors are more important than biological factors as etiological agents.
3. Seen more commonly in persons with cyclothymic temperament and melancholic personalities.	3. Seen more commonly in persons with anxious, inadequate or obsessive personalities.
4. Insomnia is of early morning type, i.e. patient wakes up by 2 a.m. or 3 a.m. and cannot sleep afterwards.	4. Insomnia is of early night type, i.e. patient finds difficulty in getting sleep, sleeps only after tossing about in the bed for long time.
5. Diurnal variation of mood present. Patient feels more miserable in morning than in evening.	5. Inverse diurnal variation of mood present; patient feels more miserable in the evening than in the morning.

Endogenous depression	Neurotic depression
6. Patient feels the same when alone or in a group.	6. Patient feels better in a group than when alone.
7. Suicidal tendencies more common.	7. Suicidal tendencies not very common.
8. Psychomotor retardation more common.	8. Psychomotor agitation, i.e. anxiety and agitation more common.
9. ECT and antidepressant drugs are the principal treatments. Psychotherapy and case work are of only supportive value.	9. Psychotherapy case work and antidepressant and antianxiety drugs are the principal treatment ECTs are not useful.

MANIA

- Mood ranging from euphoria to irritability.
- Hyper-reactivity, racing thoughts, grandiosity.
- Sleep disruption.
- Variable psychotic symptoms-paranoid ideation, gross delusion, auditory hallucination.
- Manic patients differ from schizophrenics in that the former use more effective interpersonal maneuvers, are more sensitive to social maneuvers of others and are more able to utilize weakness and vulnerability in others to their own advantage.
- *Treatment* of acute mania is (1) neuroleptics like haloperidol or olanzapine combined with benzodiazepine. The dosage of olanzapine or haloperidol is gradually reduced after lithium or another mood stabilizer is added. Clonazepam is adjunct to a neuroleptic to control acute behavioral symptoms in the dose of 1–2 mg every 4–6 hours. (2) Lithium decreases the frequency and severity of both manic and depressive attacks. Dose is 900–1200 mg daily. Moderate polyuria, polydipsia, tremor, hypothyroidism may occur and long term use may cause parkinsonian features, interstitial fibrosis and tubular atrophy. (3) Valproric acid 20 mg/kg/d, carbamazepine 800–1600 mg/d, verapamil lamotrigine

are now being used more frequently in those not responding to lithium.

INSOMNIA

- Patients may complain of difficulty in getting to sleep, or staying asleep, intermittent waking, early morning awakening or combinations of any of these. Patient may have depression, mania, alcohol abuse, heavy smoking.
- *Treatment* with lorazepam 0.5 mg, temazepam 7.5–15 mg, zolpidem 5–10 mg, zaloplon, 5–10 mg at night are effective in elderly population; twice this dose in younger patient. Short acting agents like triazolam and zolpidem may cause amnesic episodes if given regularly. Trazodone 25–150 mg at bed time is a non habit forming effective sleep medication. Diphenhydramine 25 mg or hydroxygene 25 mg at night also induce sleep.

HYPERSOMNIA

- *Narcolepsy* consists of tetrad of symptoms: (1) sudden brief sleep episodes occurring during any type of activity; (2) cataplexy – sudden loss of muscle tone; (3) sleep paralysis in full consciousness in transition period of sleep and waking; (4) hypnagogic hallucination – visual or auditory which precede sleep or occur during the sleep attack.
- *Treatment* is (a) dextroamphetamine 10 mg at morning, (b) modafinil 200 mg morning, (c) imipramine 75–100 mg daily for cataplexy but not narcolepsy.

PARASOMNIAS

- Include sleep terror, nightmares, sleep walking and enuresis. Sleep walking in elderly may be due to dementia and in adults a feature of partial complex seizure.

- *Treatment* of sleep terror, somnambulism is with diazepam 5–20 mg bed time. Enuresis is treated with imipramine 50–100 mg at bedtime or desmopression nasal spray.

ALCOHOL ABUSE/DEPENDENCY

- Physiologic dependence as evidenced from withdrawal symptoms when intake is interrupted.
- Tolerance to the effects of alcohol.
- Evidence of alcohol related diseases like alcoholic liver disease, cerebellar degeneration.
- Impairment of social and occupational functioning.
- Withdrawal symptoms are anxiety, tremulousness, mental confusion, visual hallucinations, diaphoresis, seizure (delirium tremens).
- Concurrent vitamin B_1 deficiency may cause Wernicke-Korsakoff psychosis (confusion, ataxia, ophthalmoplegia) with both anterograde and retrograde amnesia and confabulation.

Treatment

- Withdrawal symptoms treated with benzodiazepines often supplemented with clonidine 5 µg/kg, carbamazepine 400–800 mg daily, atinolol 50–100 mg daily.
- Vitamin B_1 50 mg IV, then IM daily along with pyridoxine, folic acid and Vitamin C for treatment of Wernicke-Korsakoff psychosis along with benzodiazepines.
- Maintenance of abstinence in cooperative patients with (a) disulfiram 250–500 mg daily, (b) naltrexone 50 mg daily, (c) ondasetron 4 µg/kg twice daily.

APPENDICES

- **Appendix 1**
  Conversion Formulas and Tables

- **Appendix 2**
  Blood Chemistry and laboratory Values

- **Appendix 3**
  Prescription Abbreviations

APPENDICES

APPENDIX 1

CONVERSION FORMULAS AND TABLES

CONVERSION FORMULAS

Temperature

To convert Fahrenheit to Centigrade, subtract 32 from °F, multiply by 5/9.

To convert Centigrade to Fahrenheit, multiply °C by 9/5 and add 32.

Weight

1 Kg. = 2.2 lb.	1 lb. = 0.45 kg.
1 Gm. = 15.43 grains	1 grain = 0.065 grams

Length

1 inch = 2.54 cm	1 cm = 0.3937 inch

Approximate Household Measures

1 Teaspoonful		5 cc.
1 Dessertspoonful		8 cc.
1 Tablespoonful	1/2 fl. oz	15 cc.
1 Jigger	1 1/2 fl. oz	45 cc.
1 Wineglassful	2 fl. oz	60 cc.
1 Teacupful	4 fl. oz	120 cc.
1 Glassful	8 fl. oz	240 cc.

mg. % to mEq./L

$$\frac{mg.\% \times valence \times 10}{atomic \ wt.} = mEq./L.$$

In case of gases

$$\frac{vol. \% \times 10}{22.4} = mM./L.$$

For CO_2 use 22.26 instead of 22.4

At the normal pH of body fluids, 20% of the phosphate radical is combined with one equivalent of base as BH_2PO_4 and 80% with the two equivalents of base as B_2HPO_4. Under these conditions, base equivalence per equivalent weight of 53.3 is obtained by dividing the ionic weight by 1.8 instead of by 2.

CONVERSION TABLES

Temperature

°F	°C	°C	°F
96	35.6	35.5	95.9
97	36.1	36.	96.8
98	36.7	36.5	97.9
99	37.2	37.	98.6
100	37.8	37.5	99.5
101	38.3	38.	100.4
102	38.9	38.5	101.3
103	39.4	39.	102.2
104	40.0	39.5	103.1
105	40.6	40.	104.0
106	41.1	40.5	104.9

Approximate Dosage Equivalents for Grains and Grams

Grains (gr.)	Grams (gm.)	Milligrams (mg.)
1/300	.0002	0.2
1/200	.0003	0.3
1/150	.0004	0.4
1/120	.0005	0.5
1/100	.0006	0.6
1/60	.001	1

Grains (gr.)	Grams (gm.)	Milligrams (mg.)
1/30	.002	2
1/12	.005	5
1/6	.010	10
1/4	.015	15
3/8	.025	25
1/2	.030	30
3/4	.050	50
1	.060	60
1 ½	.100	100
2	.120	120
3	.200	200
5	.300	300
7 ½	.500	500
10	.600	600
15	1	1,000
30	2	2,000
60	4	4,000

APPENDIX 2

BLOOD CHEMISTRY AND LABORATORY VALUES

BLOOD CHEMISTRY

(B-Whole Blood P-Plasma S-Serum)

Constituent	Material	mg/101. (mg.%)-or as noted I.U. = International Units I.m.U. = International Milliunits
Aldolase	S	0-6 I.mU./ml.
Aldosterone	P	7-79 mcg./100 ml.
Ammonia	P	20-150 mcg./100 ml
Amylase	S	60-160 units
(Somogyi) 0.06-0.34 I.mU./ml.		
Bilirubin – Direct	S	Up to 0.4 mg
Indirect	S	0.4-0.8 mg
Total	S	up to 1.2 mg
Bromide	S	Toxic level about 15 mEq./L
Bromosulphalein (5 mg./kg.)	S	5% dye or less at 45 minutes
Calcium	S	4.5-5.7 mEq./l
Carbon dioxide content	S	24-30 mM./L
Cephaline flocculation	S	Up to 2+ in 48 hours (Hanger)
Ceruloplasmin	S	23-50
Chloride	S	98-109 mEq./L.
Cholesterol, total		
Males, age 20-29	S	120-240 mg
30-39	S	140-270 mg
50-59	S	160-330 mg
Females lower before menopause		
Cholinesterase	S	0.5 pH unit/hour or more 2-5.3 I.U./ml.
Creatine - Males	S	0.2-0.6 mg
Females	S	0.6-1.0 mg

Constituent	Material	mg/101. (mg.%)-or as noted I.U. = International Units I.m.U. = International Milliunits
Creatine phosphokinase (CPK) = Males	S	5-50 I.MU./ml.
Females	S	5-30 I.mU./ml.
Creatinine	S	0.8-1.2 mg
Fibrinogen	P	0.2-0.4 gm./100 ml.
Glucose	S	60-100 (Nelson-Somogyi)
Glucose-6-phosphate dehydrogenase	red cells	5-10 I.U./gm. Hb./30°C.
17-Hydroxycorticosteroids		
Males	P	7-19 mcg./100 ml.
Females	P	9-21 mcg./100 ml.
After 25 units ACTH. i.m.		35-55 mcg./100 ml.
Immunoglobulins - IgG	S	800-1800 mg
IgA	S	90-450 mg
IgM	S	60-280 mg
Iodine, Protein-bound	S	4-8 mcg./100 ml.
Iron	S	50-180 mcg./100 ml.
Iron-binding capacity	S	300-360 mcg./100 ml.
17-Ketosteroids - Males	P	40-150 mcg./100 ml.
Females	P	38-130 mcg./100 ml.
Lactic Acid	B	6-20
Lactic Dehydrogenase (LDH)	S	40-60 I.m.U./ml.
Lipase	S	0.2-1.5 units/ml. (N/20 NaOH)
Lipids, total	S	400-800
cholesterol total	S	115-340
esterified	S	70%
free fatty acids	S	0.3-0.8 mEq./L
phospholipids	S	130-380
triglycerides (neutral fat)	S	10-190
Lithium (therapeutic level)	S	0.5-1.0 mEq./L
Magnesium	S	1.5-2.4 mEq./L
Non-protein nitrogen	S	25-40

Constituent	Material	mg/101. (mg.%)-or as noted I.U. = International Units I.m.U. = International Milliunits
Osmolality	S	280-290 mosm./ kg. plasma water
pH	S	7.35-7.45 glass-electrode method
Phosphatase, acid	S	0.1-1.0 units (Bodansky) 0-11 I.mU./ml.
Phosphate, akaline, Children	S	5-14 units (Bodansky) 15-20 units (King-Armstrong)
Adults	S	1.4-4.1 units (Bodansky) 4-13 units (King-Armstrong) 20-48 I.mU./ml.
Phosphorus - Children	S	2.3-3.8 mEq./L
Adults	S	1.45-2.76 mEq./L
Potassium	S	3.6-5.5 mEq./L
Proteins - Albumin	S	3.2-5.6 gm./100 ml.
α_1 Globulin	S	0.1-0.4 gm./100 ml.
α_2 Globulin	S	0.5-1.1 gm./100 ml.
β Globulin	S	0.5-1.1 gm./100 ml.
γ Globulin	S	0.5-1.6 gm./100 ml.
Salicylates (therapeutic level)	S	20-25
Sodium	S	135-145 mEq./L
Thymol turbidity	S	0-4 units (Maclagan)
Transaminase Glutamic oxalacetic (SGOT)	S	6-40 units (Karmen) 0-15 I.mU./ml.
Urea	S	17-42
Urea nitrogen	S	8-20
Uric acid - Males	S	2.1-7.8
Females	S	2.0-6.4
Zinc sulfate turbidity	S	< 12 units (Kunkel)

ELECTROPHORETIC FRACTIONS (SERUM)

Paper electrophoresis

	% of total
Albumin Globulins	45-55
α_1	5-8
α_2	8-13
β	11-17
γ	15-25

BLOOD VALUES

Haematocrit	Men : 38-54% Women : 36-47%
Hemoglobin	Men : 14-18 gm.% Women : 12-14 gm.% Children : 12-14 gm.% Newborn : 14.5-24.5 gm.%*

Blood Counts

		per cu.mm.%
Erythrocytes		
Men		$4.5\text{-}6.0 \times 10^6$
Women		$4.3\text{-}5.5 \times 10^6$
Reticulocytes		0.1%
Leukocytes, total	5000-10,000	100%
Myelocytes	0	0%
Juvenile neutrophils	0-100	0-1%
Band neutrophils	0-500	0-5%
Segmented neutrophils	2500-6000	40-60%
Lymphocytes	1000-4000	20-40%
Eosinophils	50-300	1.3%
Basophils	0-100	0-1%
Monocytes	200-800	4-8%
Platelets	200,000-500,000	

RBC Measurements

Diameter	5.5-8.8 microns (Newborn : 8.6')
Mean Corpuscular Volume	82-92 cu. microns (Newborn : 106')
Mean Corpuscular Hb (Newborn : 38')	27-31 micromicrograms
Mean Corpuscular Hb. Conc.	32-36%

Miscellaneous

Bleeding time	1-3 min. (Duke) 2-4 min. (Ivy)
Circulation time, arm to lung (either)	4-8 sec.
Circulation time arm to tongue (sodium dehydrocholate)	9-16 sec.
Clot retraction time	2-4 hrs.
Coagulation time (venous)	6-10 min. (Lee and White) 10-30 min. (Howell)
Fragility, erythrocyte (hemolysis)	0.44-0.35% NaCl
Prothrombin time	70-110% of control value
Sedimentation rate	
Men	0.9 mm. per hr. (Wintrobe)
Women	0-20 mm. per hr. (Wintrobe)

* Values for newborn are shown only where they may differ significantly from those of older children and adults.

(Whole Blood, Serum and Plasma Values)*

Acetone, serum	0.3-2 mg./100 ml.
Alpha amino nitrogen, plasma	3.5-5 mg./100 ml.
Ammonia, blood	40-70 mcg./100 ml.
Amylase, serum	80-180/Somogyi units/100 ml.
Ascorbic acid, blood	0.4-1.5 mg./100 ml.
Barbiturates, serum	0 Coma level : Phenobarbital. approximately 11 mg./100 ml.

* For some procedures, the normal values may vary according to the methods used.

	most other barbiturates
	1.5 mg./100 ml.
Base, total, serum	145-160 mEq./L.
Bilirubin, serum	
Direct	0.1-0.4 mg./100 ml.
Indirect	0.2-0.7 mg./100 ml.
	(Total minus direct)
Total	0.3-1.1 mg./100 ml.
Bromides, serum	4.5-5.5 mEq./L.
	(9-11 mg./100 mg.)
	(Slightly higher in children)
	(Varies with protein concentration)
Ionized	2.1-2.6 mEq./L.
	(4.25-5.25 mg./100 ml.)
Carbon dioxide, serum	
Content	26-28 mEq./L.
	Infants: 20-26 mEq./L.
Combining power 24-29	(53-64 vol%)
mEq./L.	
Tension, pCO_2	35-45 mm. Hg
Carbon monoxide, blood	Symptoms with over 20%
	saturation
Carotenoids, serum	100-300 I.U./100 ml.
Chloride, serum	100-106 mEq./L.
	(355-376 mg./100 ml. as Cl)
	(585-620 mg./100 ml. as NaCl) .
Cholestrol serum	
Total	150-250 mg./100 ml.
Esters	68-76% of total cholestrol
Copper, serum	70-140 mg./100 ml.
Creatinine, serum	0.7-1.5 mg./100 ml.
Cryoglobulins, serum	0
Dilatin blood or serum	Therapeutic levels :
	1-11 mcg./ml.
Ethanol, blood	
Marked intoxication	0.3-0.4%
Alcoholic stupor	0.4-0.5%
Coma	Above 0.5%
Fibrinogen, plasma	200-400 mg./100 ml.
Glucose (fasting), blood	
True	60-100 mg./100 ml.
Folin	80-120 mg./100 ml.

17-Hydroxycorticoids, plasma	5-25 mcg./100 ml.
Icterus index, serum	4-7
Iodine, butanol extractable serum	3.5-6.5 mcg./100 ml.
Iodine, protein-bound, serum	3.5-8 mcg./100 ml. (may be slightly higher in infants)
Iron, serum	75-175 mcg./100 ml.
Iron-binding capacity, unsaturated, serum	150-300 mcg./100 ml.
Lactic acid, blood	6-16 mg./100 ml.
Lactic dehydrogenase, serum	200-450 units/100 ml.
Lead, blood	0.50 mcg./100 ml.
Lipase, serum	Less than 1.5 units (ml, of Nl 20 NaOH)
Lipids, total, serum	450-850 mg./100 ml.
Lipid partition, blood	
Cholestrol	150-250 mg./100 ml.
Cholestrol esters	68-76% of total cholestrol
Phospholipids	6-12 mg./100 ml. as lipid phosphorus
Total fatty acids	190-420 mg./100 ml.
Neutral fat	0-150 mg./100 ml.
Magnesium, serum	1.5-2.5 mEq./L/ (1.8-3 mg/100 ml.)
Nitrogen, nonprotein, serum	15-35 mg./100 ml.
Osmolality, serum	285-295 mOsm./L.
Oxygen, blood	
Capacity	16-24 vol.% (varies with Hb)
Content	
Arterial	15-23 vol.%
Venous	10-16 vol.%
Saturation	
Arterial	94-100% of capacity
Venous	60-85% of capacity
Tension, PO_2	
Arterial	95-100 mm.Hg
pH, arterial, plasma	7.35-7.45
Phenylalanine, serum	Less than 3 mg./100 ml.
Phosphatase, acid, serum	1-5 units (King-Armstrong) 0.5-2 units (Bodansky) 0.5-2 units (Gutman) 0.1-1 units (Shinowara) 0.10.63 units (Bessey-Lowry)

Phosphate, alkaline, serum	5-13 units (King-Armstrong)
	2-4.5 units (Bodansky)
	3-10 units (Gutman)
	2.2-8.6 units (Shinowara)
	0.8-2.3 units (Bessey-Lowry)
	(Values are higher in children)
Phosphate, inorganic, serum	2-4.5 mg./100 ml.
	(Children : 4-7 mg./100 ml.
Potassium, serum	3.5-5 mEq./L.
	(14-20 mg./100 ml. as K)
Proteins, serum	
Total	6-8 gm./100 ml.
Albumin	3.5-5.5 gm./100 ml.
Globulin	1.5-3 gm./100 ml.
Paper electrophoresis	
Albumin	45-55% of total
Globulin	
α_1	5-8% of total
α_2	8-13% of total
β	11-17% of total
γ	15-25% of total
Pyruvic acid, plasma	1.2 mg./100 ml.
Salicylate, plasma	0
Therapeutic range	20-25 mg./100 ml.
Toxic range	Over 30 mg./100 ml.
Serotonin	
Platelet suspension	0.1-0.3 mcg./ml. blood
Serum	0.1-0.32 mcg./ml.
Sodium, serum	136-145 mEq./L.
	(313-334 mg./100 ml. as Na)
Sulfates, inorganic, serum	0.5-1.5 mg./100 ml.
Transaminase, serum	0.5-1.5 mg./100 ml.
SGOT	5-40 units/ml.
SGPT	5-35 units/ml.
Urea nitrogen, blood (BUN)	10-20 mg./100 ml.
Uric acid, serum	3-6 mg./100 ml.
Vitamin A, serum	30-100 units/100 ml.

NORMAL URINE VALUES

Acetone and acetoacetate	0
Addiscount	
Erythrocytes	0-130, 000/24 hr.

Leukocytes	0-650,000/24 hr.
Casts (hyaline)	0-2,000/24 hr.
Aldosterone	2-23 mcg./24 hr.
Alpha amino nitrogen	64-199 mg./24 hr.
	(Not over 1.5% total nitrogen)
Ammonia	20-70 mEq./L.
Amylase (Somogyi)	260-950 Somogyi units/24 hr.
Calcium	
Low Ca diet (Bauer-Aub)	Less than 150 mg./24 hr.
Usual diet	Less than 250 mg./24 hr.
Catecholamines	
Epinephrine	Less than 10 mcg./24 hr.
Norepinephrine	Less than 100 mcg./24 hr.
Chorionic gonadotropin	0
Coproporphyrin	50-250 mcg./24 hr.
	(Higher in children and during pregnancy)
Creatinine	15-25 mg./Kg. body wt./24 hr.
Cystine or cysteine	0
Estrogens	
Male	4-25 mcg./24 hr.
Female	4-60 mcg./24 hr.
	(Increased during pregnancy)
Hemoglobin and Myoglobin	0
Homogentisic acid	0
5-Hydroxyindolylacetic acid (5-HIAA)	
Qualitative	0
Quantitative	Less than 16 mg./24 hr.
17-Hydroxycorticoids	
Male	5-15 mg./24 hr.
Female	4-10 mg./24 hr.
	(Varies with method used)
17-Ketosteroids	
Under 8 years	0-2 mg./24 hr.
Adolescents	2-20 mg./24 hr.
Male	8-25 mg./24 hr.
Female	5-15 mg./24 hr.
	Lead Less than 0.08 mcg./ml. or less than 120 mcg./24 hr.
pH	4.8-8; average 6 (depends on diet)

Phenylpyruvic acid	0
Pituitary gonadotropins	5-10 rat units/24 hr.
	10-50 mouse units/24 hr.
	(increased after menopause)
Porphobilinogen	0
Protein	0 qualitative
	(Less than 30 mg./24 hr.)
Specific gravity	30-70 gm./L; average
Solids, total	50 gm./L/ (To estimate total solids per liter, multiply last two figures of specific gravity by 2.66, Long's coefficient)
Sugar	0
Titratable acidity	20-40 mEq./24 hr.
Urobilinogen	Up to 1 Ehrlich unit/2 hr. (1-3 p.m.)
	0-4 mg./24 hr.
Vanillylmandelic acid (VMA)	1.8-8.4 mg./24 hr.

URINE

Specific gravity : 1.015-1.025
pH : 6 (4.8-8.0)
Volume : 1200 (600-2500) ml./24 hr.
Night vol./Day. vol. = 1 : 2 to 1 : 4
Night urine-less than 700 ml.; Sp, gr. greater than 1.018
Total solids : 55-70 gm./24 hr.

The output of electrolytes and inorganic elements is a function of the diet.

Constituent	24-Hour Excretion or as noted
Aldosterone	2-23 jmcq.
Ammonia	20-70 mEq.
acid loading	70-100 mEq.
Amylase	260-950 mg. glucose
Calcium	5-12.5 mEq.
	(average diet)
	12.5-15 mEq.
	(high calcium diet)

Catecholamines	
Epinephrine	under 10 mcg.
Norepinephrine	under 100 mcg.
Chloride	110-250 mEq.
Creatine	
Males	0-40 mg.
Females	0-100 mg.
Higher in children and during pregnancy	
Creatinine	5-15 mg/Kg.
Estriol-pregnancy	
Week	Range
16	up to 3 mg.
20	1-9 mg.
24	4-12 mg.
28	5-17 mg.
32	6-22 mg.
36	8-32 mg.
40	9-37 mg.
Estrogen	
Males	4-25 mcg.
Females	4-60 mcg.
5-HIAA	< 16 mg.
17-Hydroxycorticosteroids	
Males	5.5-14.5 mg.
Females	4.9-12.9 mg.
After 25 units ACTH (i.m.)	200-400% increase
17-Ketosteroids	
Males	8-15 mg.
Females	6-11.5 mg.
Children	
< 12 years	< 5 mg.
12-15 years	5-12 mg.
After 25 units ACTH (i.m.)	50-100% increase
Lead	100-1000 mcg.
Osmolality	300-1000 mOsm./kg. water-varies with diet and fluid intake
Phosphorus inorganic	0.78-1.1 gm. (average diet)
Potassium	25-100 mEq.

Pregnanediol	
Children	negative
Males	0-1 mg.
Females	
Proliferative phase	0.5-1.5 mg.
Luteal phase	2-8 mg.
Postmenopausal	0.2-1 mg.
Peak during	
pregnancy	60-100 mg.
Protein (albumin)	10-100 mg.
Sodium	130-260 mEq.
Urea nitrogen	6-17 gm.
Uric acid	0.2-0.7 gm.
Urobilinogen	0.1-1 Ehrlich unit/100 ml.
Uroporphyrin	10-30 mcg.
VMA up to 9 mg.	

STOOL

Fat	
Total	10-25% and <5 gm./24 hr.
Neutral	1-5% of dry matter
Free fatty acids	5-13% of dry matter
Combined fatty acids	5-15% of dry matter
Urobilinogen	40-200 mg./24 hr.

KIDNEY FUNCTION TESTS

Constituent or Factor	Normal Values	Remarks
Endogenous Creatinine Clearance (glomerular filtration primarily). As creatinine blood level rises a greater volume of urine is secreted by the tubules.	With normal physical activity 90-130 ml./min. per 1.73 sq. meters body surface.	Calculated from concentration of substance in urine and plasma, and the proportion excreted per min.

Constituent or Factor	Normal Values	Remarks
Inulin Clearance (glomerular filtration exclusively).	Male : 130±20 Female :120±15 ml./min. per 1.73 sq.meters body surface	Short duration test Administered intravenously
Urea Clearance (glomerular filtration and partial tubular reabsorption).	Maximum : 60-90 ml. per minute Standard : 60-90 ml. per minute	Calculated number of ml.blood completely cleared of urea as blood passes through kidneys during 1 min.; diuresis over 2 ml./min.
Phenolsulfonph- thalein (chiefly tubular secretion, partially glomerular filtration)	25% or more in 15 min. 40-60% in 1 hr. 60-85% in 2 hr.	Administered intra- venously. Since tubular transport mechanism is not saturated by dose used, the test mainly a reflection of renal blood flow.
Concentration and Dilution	Sp. gr. 1.025- 1.032 concentration) Sp. gr. 1.001- 1.003 (dilution)	After fluids withheld for 10 hr. or more Administer 1500 ml. of water. It is totally excreted in 2-4 hr., most during 1st hr.
Diodrast Clearance (effective renal plasma flow and tubular function)	Male : 600-800 Female : 500-700 ml./min. per 1.73 sq meters body surface	Rapidly and actively secreted by renal tubules
p-Aminohippurate Clearance (effective renal plasma flow and tubular function	Male : 600-800 Female : 500-700 ml./min. per 1.73 sq meters body surface	Rapidly and actively secreted by renal tubuler

APPENDIX 3

PRESCRIPTION ABBREVIATIONS

aa (ana)	–	of each (equal parts)
a.c. (ante cibum)	–	before meals
aq. (aqua)	–	water
b.i.d. (bis in die)	–	twice a day
caps. (capsula)	–	capsule
Chart (chartulae)	–	papers (powders)
ft. (fiat)	–	make
h.s. (hora somni)	–	at bed time
M. (misce)	–	mix
m.dict. (modo dictu)	–	as directed
non rep.	–	do not repeat
(non repetatur)		(do not refill)
o.d. (oculus dexter)	–	right eye
o.s. (oculus sinister)	–	left eye
p.c. (post cibum)	–	after meals
p.r.n. (pro re nata)	–	as needed
q.h. (quaque hora)	–	every hour
q.i.d. (quates in die)	–	four time a day
q.s. (quantum sufficit)	–	a sufficient quantity
R_x (recipe)	–	take (thou) a recipe
sig. (signa)	–	write on label
stat. (statim)	–	immediately
t.i.d. (ter in die)	–	three times a day
ut dict. (ut dictum)	–	as directed
gr.	–	grain or grains
gtt. (gutta/e)	–	drop(s)
m.	–	minim
ℨiss	–	one and one-half drams
ℨ +	–	one ounce
ℨ ss	–	one-half ounce
cc.	–	cubic centimeter
gm.	–	gram
mg.	–	milligram
mcg	–	microgram
ml.	–	milliliter

Index

D

E

F

G

H

Haemolytic uremic syndrome (HUS) *197*
Haemorrhoids *170*
Hairy cell leukemia *193*
Hantavirus syndrome *7*
Hepatic steatosis (fatty liver) *175*
Hepatobiliary diseases *171*
Hepatocellular carcinoma *179*
Herpes encephalitis *145*
Herpes simplex *1*
Hirsutism and virilization *68*
Histoplasmosis *38*
Hodgkin's lymphoma *195*
Hyperaldosteronism *69*
Hypercalcemia *209*
Hyperkalemia *208*
Hypermagnesemia *210*
Hypernatremia *208*
Hyperparathyroidism *65*
Hyperprolactinemia *61*
Hypersensitive pneumonitis *96*
Hypersomnia *237*
Hyperthyroidism *63*
Hypertrophic cardiomyopathy *106*
Hypocalcemia *209*
Hypokalemia *208*
Hypomagnesemia *210*
Hyponatremia *207*
Hypoparathyroidism *65*
Hypophosphatemia *210*
Hypopituitarism *59*
Hypotension *224*
Hypothermia *223*
Hypothyroidism *62*

I

Idiopathic thrombocytopenic purpura (ITP) *196*
Impetigo *217*
Infectious diseases *1*
Infectious esophagitis *153*
Infectious mononucleosis *3*
Influenza *9*
Insomnia *237*
Interstitial cystitis *55*

Interstitial lung disease *91*
Interstitial nephritis *51*
Intestinal tuberculosis *163*
Intracerebral haemorrhage *128*
Intracranial tumors *131*
Iron deficiency anaemia *185*
Irritable bowel syndrome (IBS) *163*

K

Kawasaki syndrome *10*

L

Legionnaire's disease *16*
Leishmaniasis *25*
Leptospirosis *24*
Lichen planus *214*
Lichen simplex (neurodermatitis) *213*
Listeriosis *15*
Loiasis *37*
Lower GI bleed *150*
Lyme disease *24*
Lymphocytic choriomeningitis *145*

M

Maduromycosis *40*
Malabsorption *161*
Malaria *41*
Male hypogonadism *70*
Mania *236*
Measles *4*
Medullary sponge kidney *52*
Megaloblastic anaemia *186*
Metabolic acidosis *211*
Methanol and ethylene glycol *226*
Migraine *121*
Motor neurone disease *138*
Mucocutaneous candidiasis *219*
Mucormycosis *40*
Multinodular goiter *62*
Multiple myeloma *195*
Multiple sclerosis (MS) *137*
Mumps *4*
Myasthenia gravis *140*
Mycosis fungoides (cutaneous T cell lymphoma) *216*